PERFORMANCE AND IMAGE ENHANCING DRUGS AND SUBSTANCES

In the pursuit of more muscle, enhanced strength, sustained endurance and idealised physiques, an increasing number of elite athletes, recreational sport enthusiasts and body-conscious gym-users are turning to performance and image enhancing drugs and substances (PIEDS). In many instances, such use occurs with little regard for the health, social and economic consequences.

This book presents a nuanced, evidence-based examination of PIEDS. It provides a classification of PIEDS types, physical impacts, rates of use, user profiles, legal and sporting status, and remedial programme interventions, covering both elite and recreational use.

It offers the perfect guide to assist students, government policy makers and sport managers in understanding the complex issues surrounding PIEDS consumption.

Aaron C. T. Smith is Professor of Sport Business at the Institute for Sport Business, Loughborough University London, UK. His research investigates psychological, organisational and policy change in sport, business, health, religion, technology and society.

Bob Stewart is a Principle Consultant with Aztek Developments and a former Professor of Sport Policy in the College of Sport and Exercise Science at Victoria University, Australia. Bob has a special interest in player regulation in professional team sports, and the ways in which the forces of neoliberalism and hyper-commercialism shape the structure and conduct of contemporary sport.

Kate Westberg is Associate Professor of Marketing at RMIT University, Australia. Her research focuses primarily on the areas of sport marketing and sponsorship, branding, social marketing and behavioural change.

Constantino Stavros is Associate Professor of Marketing at RMIT University, Australia, and the Editor-in-Chief of *Sport, Business and Management: An International Journal*. His research interests lie predominantly at the intersection of consumption and technology.

PERFORMANCE AND IMAGE ENHANCING DRUGS AND SUBSTANCES

Issues, Influences and Impacts

*Aaron C. T. Smith, Bob Stewart,
Kate Westberg and
Constantino Stavros*

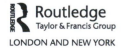

Routledge
Taylor & Francis Group

LONDON AND NEW YORK

First published 2018
by Routledge
2 Park Square, Milton Park, Abingdon, Oxon OX14 4RN

and by Routledge
711 Third Avenue, New York, NY 10017

Routledge is an imprint of the Taylor & Francis Group, an informa business

© 2018 Aaron C. T. Smith, Bob Stewart, Kate Westberg and Constantino Stavros

The right of Aaron C. T. Smith, Bob Stewart, Kate Westberg and Constantino Stavros to be identified as authors of this work has been asserted by them in accordance with sections 77 and 78 of the Copyright, Designs and Patents Act 1988.

British Library Cataloguing-in-Publication Data
A catalogue record for this book is available from the British Library

Library of Congress Cataloging-in-Publication Data
A catalog record for this book has been requested

ISBN: 978-1-138-49294-3 (hbk)
ISBN: 978-1-138-49295-0 (pbk)
ISBN: 978-1-351-02934-6 (ebk)

Typeset in Bembo and Stone Sans
by Florence Production Ltd, Stoodleigh, Devon, UK

CONTENTS

DISCLAIMER

This book contains general information about medical conditions, drugs and symptoms. The information is not advice, and should not be treated as such. The contents of this book are not a substitute for independent professional advice and are not intended to diagnose, treat, cure or prevent any disease, nor should they be used for therapeutic purposes or as a substitute for a health professional's advice.

ACKNOWLEDGEMENT

The research reported in this book was supported by the Alcohol and Drug Foundation, Australia.

1

APPLY, INGEST, INJECT AND REGRET

Introduction to performance and image enhancing substances

Introduction: Overview of the book

More than a billion people apply, ingest or inject performance and image enhancing drugs and substances (PIEDS) daily to swell muscle mass, shed fat, sustain endurance, resist fatigue, stimulate energy, improve mood, tolerate pain, deflate inflammation, enhance relaxation, promote concentration, sharpen reactions, maintain alertness, reduce fluid, control steadiness, augment body shape, induce euphoria and strengthen confidence.[1] PIEDS are used to make us look and feel better. The dilemma is, however, that better-looking and -feeling bodies now can come with regret later.

Our aim in this book is to present an easy-to-understand summary and review of the implications associated with the use of PIEDS. We therefore view this book as a 'primer'—a concentrated guide to understanding PIEDS. It is not a 'user's guide'. Rather, this primer focuses on educating and informing anyone interested in PIEDS by identifying the risks associated with their use, from the likelihood of wasting money on ineffective supplements, to the potential for serious harm. However, the forthcoming content should not be seen as a medical guide, or a definitive assessment of each PIEDS type. Many of the PIEDS reviewed here remain under-researched, the full implications of their long-term use unknown. As a result, a comprehensive evaluation cannot be undertaken, so readers should approach the content aware that in many cases the best we can provide is an introductory overview. We advise every reader to consult a medical professional prior to using any PIEDS.

While elite and professional sports have become inexorably linked with performance enhancing drugs, the full extent of their use across the sporting and general community remains unknown. As this book notes, however, the use of substances for image enhancing purposes has escalated to the extent that the volume and scope of use overshadows that within sport's elite ranks. The unregulated use of PIEDS presently constitutes a serious health and social concern.

This book observes the rise of PIEDS alongside their more ready accessibility, a combination that has enticed almost everyone physically active to test out one form of PIEDS or another, from legal, health-bolstering supplements to illicit, health-risky pharmaceuticals. PIEDS are no longer just the purview of elite athletes.

This book contains seven chapters. Chapter 1, here, continues with a summary of the primer's 10 key conclusions. These are: 1) The abuse of some PIEDS can have serious, deleterious implications for the long-term health of users, both during active use and well after use has discontinued. 2) The use of PIEDS exclusively for image enhancing purposes now exceeds PIEDS use for sporting performance or for medical interventions. 3) Most PIEDS usage is moderate, but the pathological and supra-therapeutic use of substances, dosages and combinations has become normalised in some communities. 4) PIEDS users obtain a significant amount of their knowledge and advice about substances, effects, dosages and distribution through unreliable online sources. 5) The authenticity, quality and potential contamination of PIEDS products have become worrisome. 6) The majority of pharmaceutical-grade PIEDS are acquired without medical guidance or a prescription. 7) Driving forces behind PIEDS use include gender associations, dysfunctional body images and a powerful desire to meet the cultural ideals of health and image. 8) More effective programmes for changing attitudes, behaviours or intentions relating to PIEDS deliver over longer periods, comprise numerous teaching sessions, address a range of topics including drug- and alcohol-related issues and alternatives to drug use and media/peer pressure resistance, and increase participant involvement and ownership through peer-led teaching. 9) Emerging evidence links PIEDS abuse with gateway behaviours, beginning with dietary and nutritional supplements (DNS) and moving into performance enhancing drugs (PEDS). 10) There remains a great deal of confusion about the effects, veracity, risks and legality of different PIEDS.

The remainder of this chapter introduces the problems and issues associated with PIEDS use. It outlines some foundational influences related to PIEDS use, such as their relationship to a user's life course and the possibility that certain substances serve as gateways to others. Our review demonstrates the need for more research examining the decision-making driving use, as well as the contextual, experiential and behavioural pathways that shape these decisions. Not only must we better understand what influences decisions to employ PIEDS, but we also need to provide policy makers with solid data about how decisions may be influenced in order to produce more responsible practices in the future. Sport and health policy makers need avenues to help users mark out substance-use boundaries that protect their personal health and well-being, without constraining them from improving their physical performances and general health. We suggest that the conclusions noted in this book are important because the decision to use PIEDS can lead to health risks.

Chapter 2 examines the nature, types and use of dietary and nutritional supplements (DNS) as PIEDS. DNS are not inherently unhealthy products in the same way that alcohol, sugary drinks and fast foods may be considered unhealthy.

However, concerns have been raised with respect to their efficacy, health risks and the potential for accidental doping. While the efficacy of supplements remains difficult to ascertain, meta-analyses of commonly sold supplements have generally come to the conclusion that while some are demonstrably efficacious, a large percentage of the market consists of products with little or no scientific backing. This is significant because not only do supplement companies promote specifically sports-associated supplements (such as creatine, energy bars, etc.), but they also promote various sport- or health-related products (vitamins, daily health-boosting products, etc.). Evidently some products do have benefits, but the current evidence is not of sufficient quality from which informed decisions can be made. While elite athletes and coaches might be highly knowledgeable about which products to use and when, the general public is unlikely to have access to detailed scientific data on product efficacy or applicability to their exercise and/or health requirements.

With respect to the health risks of DNS use, while acute adverse effects are uncommon there are some indications that the use of some supplements may result in unwelcome health outcomes. Nevertheless, this is rare and usually associated with substances now prohibited in sport, or with excessive dosages. Perhaps more worrying is the skewed perception that all DNS products are safe to take in any amount. Another concern with respect to DNS is that they may contain prohibited, unlabelled substances. While not a concern for the majority of people taking DNS, it may be relevant for elite-amateur or semi-professional athletes.

Chapter 3 explores the scale and scope of PIEDS use. The scope, magnitude and diversity of substance use in sport and recreation make its study complex. For example, some substance use is common, benign and even advantageous to health. Such usage includes the infrequent use of painkillers, the moderate consumption of coffee and the liberal use of most vitamins and recovery supplements such as protein powders. At the same time, both serious recreational athletes and elite athletes use a range of additional substances, the health implications of which range from the uncertain to the severely dangerous. Examples of the latter include the use of significant quantities of analgesics, stimulants, anabolic agents or hormones, sometimes combined in experimental cocktails and dosages. In some cases, athletes employ pharmaceutical products designed for use with animals, while in other cases they test out the latest—probably ineffectual—designer nutritional supplements.

In short, a huge variety of PIEDS are available for athletes to ingest or inject. Adding to the uncertainty is the combination of widespread availability—often through Internet-order mail—and limited (or no) regulation ensuring security around the quality, efficacy and legality of the PIEDS. Since most athletes, both recreational and elite, self-prescribe PIEDS, they tend to engage in potentially dangerous practices such as the ingestion of high dosages, failure to cycle off or in lower dosages, the use of experimental substances, the use of untried combinations and the unknowing use of tainted, contaminated, mislabelled and inauthentic substances, all the while receiving advice on use from a variety of different-quality sources such as coaches, peers, supplement marketers or web forums.

Chapter 4 considers the impact of culture, values and ethnicity on PIEDS use. The evidence indicates that PIEDS use has permeated throughout all cultures and contexts. Alarmingly, it begins in school sport, although most of the available data come from American high schools where inter-school sport is highly valued, and where it contributes significantly to a school's reputation and financial viability. PIEDS use also seems prevalent in community gyms and fitness centres, with Europe and the United States (US) featuring prominently. Substances of all kinds appear liberally in US colleges and universities as well, where both licit and illicit substance use is usually higher amongst athletes than non-athletes. Irrespective of some minor differences, the studies show that people of all backgrounds who play sport regularly hang around sport clubs, use gyms to build their bodies and do actually use PIEDS more often than those who pursue other leisure activities.

Chapter 5 offers a review of PIEDS that can be employed for cognitive enhancement. It concludes that cognitive enhancers may only provide modest improvements to memory or decision-making. In fact, some evidence highlights the potential for cognitive enhancers to reduce cognitive efficiency, and may actually prove deleterious to athletes seeking to make rapid decisions. Given that the empirical examination of cognitive boosters remains nascent, much work needs to be undertaken to determine whether their use delivers any performance enhancement and/or constitutes a health concern.

Chapter 6 provides a typology of PIEDS classes and effects, based on three main strata, Dietary and Nutritional Supplements (DNS), Enhancement & Augmentation (EA) and Performance Enhancing Drugs (PEDS). DNS have been further sub-categorised into four types of effects: 1) Power & Muscle; 2) Energy & Endurance; 3) Fat & Metabolism; and 4) Immunity & Inflammation. EA comprises a single category, labelled number '5'. PEDS encompasses 10 sub-categories, '6–15': 6) Anabolic Agents; 7) Hormones; 8) Hormone Manipulators; 9) Beta-2 Agonists; 10) Masking Agents; 11a) Stimulants; 11b) Cognitive Enhancers; 12) Pain & Pleasure Narcotics; 13) Adrenal Manipulators; 14) Psychoactives; and 15) Anti-inflammatories. A summary matrix is provided for each sub-category of PIEDS containing information about its nature, effects and risk profile.

Finally, Chapter 7 reviews the key points made in the book and summarises the impact of PIEDS through a performance-based typology and a PIEDS effects map. In the following section, the book's critical arguments and findings are compiled and explained.

Summary of key points

We define PIEDS as any material that an individual enters (through ingestion or injection) into, or applies on the surface of his or her body, to enhance physical or cognitive performance and/or appearance. Included are pharmaceutical drugs and dietary or nutritional supplements. PIEDS also encompass any substance used for augmenting aesthetic bodily appearance. Included are substances that athletes use for recreational, recovery or stress-management purposes, and which may be perceived as indirectly performance enhancing. These substances may also take the form of 'nootropics', or so-called 'smart' drugs, which are perceived to deliver cognitive enhancements in the form of improved focus, concentration, alertness and rapid decision-making.

We conclude that the misuse and abuse of some PIEDS presents an increasing health problem.[2] Although the evidence remains nascent, several alarming issues and trends foreshadow a worsening in PIEDS-related physical and social harms. We present 10 major findings.

The first finding confirms the medical consensus that the abuse of some PIEDS can have serious, negative effects upon the long-term health of users, both during active use and well after use has discontinued. In fact, the abuse of certain PIEDS—especially those of pharmaceutical grade such as anabolic androgenic steroids (AAS) and hormones—have been connected to a greater risk of death, as well as a confronting array of cardiovascular, psychiatric, metabolic, endocrine, neurological, infectious, hepatic, renal and musculoskeletal disorders.[3] To make matters more alarming, we note that a large majority of non-pharmaceutical PIEDS—what are mainly dietary and nutritional supplements (DNS)—are poorly understood, with little evidence available to substantiate their claims of inducing a measurable effect on the body. Although the abuse of some DNS can incur undesirable health effects, only a small group of DNS can be confidently said to have a trivial to moderate positive impact. Most, however, are unlikely to do anything at all other than lighten a wallet or purse.

The second finding highlights that the use of PIEDS exclusively for image enhancing purposes has grown so much that it now exceeds PIEDS use for either sporting performance or medical interventions. Image enhancing here refers to the use of PIEDS for body shaping or other recreational, cosmetic or occupational reasons.[4] Despite media-fuelled perceptions that PIEDS use is a problem associated with elite sport that has to do with cheating rather than health, the reality is that the majority of users are non-athletes who are unknowingly placing their health at serious risk.[5] A recent study corroborated that PIEDS use can be motivated by appearance, improved health and dysfunctional body image just as much, if not more often, than superior sport performance.[6] A UK survey concluded that over 70% of AAS users were motivated by bodybuilding alone.[7] Similarly, an Australian study identified several principle PIEDS user groups in addition to serious sports-people, including occupational users from protective services and entertainment industries, body image users and adolescents.[8]

Although less intuitive, it seems premature to conclude that the problem only lies with younger men. In fact, the epidemic-like inflation of obesity—combined with the ubiquitous display of idealised, youthful bodies in the mainstream media—has created a new contingent of body conscious older adults who worry and stress about their body images.[9] However, unlike previous generations whose budgets were tight, these older, increasingly image-conscious groups have available to them a vast suite of PIEDS, and a surfeit of disposable income to throw at their body problems. Throughout this book we repeatedly observe the absence of research investigating the use of substances by older people who are pursuing the primary aim of enhancing appearance. It would be premature to assume that all women want to look slim and all men muscular, or that gender is the most important factor in a given individual's 'embodied motivations'.[10] However, it also is clear that relatively older women and men may have similar levels of body dissatisfaction to younger people.[11] For example, a recent study by Gough et al.[12] showed that overweight men, including some in their 60s, reported high levels of body dissatisfaction.

A third finding goes beyond the scope of singular use, and reflects a newly firming level of use that involves untested and supra-therapeutic substances, dosages and combinations. While studies show that most usage is moderate, researchers have revealed that pathological use has become normalised in some PIEDS communities.[13] For example, one large study on AAS reported that bodybuilding users consumed supra-physiologic (above the natural amount found in the body) doses, and combined these casually with other substances. These recreational users practised experimental poly-pharmacy and had a higher than usual likelihood of meeting the criteria for substance dependence disorder.[14] Other studies have further revealed that AAS users combine multiple drugs in volumes that are 10–100-fold the pharmacological dosage for testosterone deficiency. This practice is colloquially known as 'stacking', with substances taken orally, injected or, more commonly, both. Mixing two or more substances in the same syringe has also become sufficiently common to attract its own nomenclature—'blending'.[15] Experimental combinations, or 'stacks', amplify the risk of negative substance interactions where one or more of the compounds counter-indicate another ingredient. In addition, emerging research has pointed to a unique profile of users, health effects and sourcing approaches associated with methods of appearance modification, especially by injecting non-pharmaceutical substances. The consumers using these methods do not identify as 'drug users' and tend to be poorly informed about the risks of injection practices such as contamination and needle sharing. They also rely on the Internet to obtain information and access to augmentation products.[16]

A fourth finding indicates that PIEDS users obtain a significant amount of their knowledge and advice about substances, effects, dosages and distribution through unreliable online sources. Sometimes referred to as 'lifestyle drugs', the range of PIEDS available online cater for every imaginable sexual, muscular, cognitive and natural capacity. This is a new and fast-growing trend of abuse that needs further investigation. One study conducted with (non-medical) PIEDS (mainly AAS) users reported that 62% had sought information from Internet sites and 55% from friends.[17] As the researchers concluded, an over-reliance on web forums and personal networks compromises the quality of advice offered to users about everything from substance effects to primary care services. Other studies have highlighted the prevalence of forums dedicated to discussing and sharing guidelines for PIEDS use, especially AAS.[18] Thousands of sites can be readily located. Most take strong pro-drug positions and undermine the legitimacy of medical advice and knowledge. They also offer a raft of PIEDS for sale, along with recommendations on dosages and effective combinations with other PIEDS.[19]

A fifth finding relates to the authenticity, quality and potential contamination of PIEDS products. As AAS have become synonymous with low-effort, high-muscle physiques, stimulants and hormones have radically increased in popularity to reduce fat for a chiselled but diet-free body. Of course, these substances were originally developed for therapeutic use but have been re-purposed for human enhancements. Adding to well-known substances are an assortment of new and specialised drugs (some popular ones are equine veterinary products), about which little is known.[20] Ready availability via the Internet has also encouraged users to experiment with what were once prohibitively expensive and powerful substances, such as human growth hormone (hGH). However, even though genuine hGH remains too costly for all but the professional athlete or the obsessed, mail order providers promise vastly cheaper synthetic versions that can contain a wide variety of non-hGH concoctions. In one sample obtained from the 'underground' market, 53% of the injectable AAS and 21% of the oral tablets were counterfeit.[21] Even worse, the samples contained bacterial organisms likely to create skin abscesses at the injection site.

The illicit manufacture of PIEDS raises concerns about quality and sterility, bacterial contamination and whether the contents actually match the label.[22] Another study taking an in-depth look at the authenticity of the cognitive enhancer, Piracetam, concluded that the health risks were elevated given the significant chance that the products sold online might be counterfeits.[23] Furthermore, studies on nutritional supplements have revealed the undeclared presence of substances such as ephedrine and its analogues (pseudoephedrine), caffeine, 3,4-methylene-dioxy-N-methylamphetamine (MDMA, or 'ecstasy') and other amphetamine-related compounds.[24] Our analysis highlights evidence (reported in the forthcoming PIEDS summary matrices) that the contamination issue is a particular concern for imported supplements.

Following on from the previous issue concerning quality, a sixth finding relates to the volume of pharmaceutical-grade PIEDS reportedly acquired without medical guidance or a prescription.[25] To make matters worse, studies have shown that most of the PIEDS used without a prescription were not manufactured by pharmaceutical companies under quality-controlled conditions.[26] Considering the vast range of pharmaceutical-grade PIEDS used for performance and image purposes, the combination of quality uncertainty and dosage/administration irregularities creates a dangerous collision.[27] In addition to the prevalence of PIEDS manufactured illegally in underground laboratories and potentially containing any number of toxic or filler contaminants, the most serious image enhancers use veterinary-grade pharmaceuticals.[28]

A seventh finding relates to the gender associations and dysfunctional body image perceptions underpinning PIEDS abuse. We uncovered a growing amount of evidence exposing a desire to meet cultural ideals of health and image.[29] According to body image experts, adolescents, and especially young men, have become increasingly and obsessively preoccupied by the muscularity of their appearance in a form of distorted perception known as 'muscle dysmorphia'.[30] Young men displaying muscle dysmorphia describe an intense dissatisfaction with their body size and shape because they perceive themselves as being inadequately muscled. Not only does muscle dysmorphia stimulate PIEDS abuse, it also corresponds to higher levels of mood disorders, anxiety, obsessive compulsive behaviours and other forms of social impairment.[31]

Numerous studies have revealed that most males expressing muscle dysmorphia engage in bodybuilding practices and consume copious quantities of dietary and nutritional supplements. Around half reported a lifetime use of AAS.[32] Not only has AAS use been associated with negative body image, but men whose use is driven by appearance or image concerns have been revealed as a particularly dysfunctional subgroup.[33] As a result, male bodybuilders—whether recreational or professional—are at a higher risk for body image pathologies. They also present similar psychological characteristics to those suffering from eating disorders, which in turn predicts AAS use in males.[34] High levels of stimulant use in Brazil, for example, have been attributed to ubiquitous self-administration and a 'body shaping' culture.[35]

An eighth finding shows the absence of effective educational interventions concerning PIEDS and their safe consumption. There appears to be an almost unequivocal consensus that the use of PIEDS is growing outside elite and organised sporting systems, and that the misuse of such substances in recreational and community sport represents an urgent social and public health issue. Little is known, however, about what constitutes best practice in this area given the limited attention and study that has been undertaken both outside the US and in the context of community and recreational sporting participation. Overall it appears that programmes which are somewhat effective in changing attitudes, behaviours or intentions relating to PIEDS have the following characteristics: a) delivery over longer periods (2–10 weeks) and comprise a number of teaching sessions rather than delivered on a 'one shot' basis; b) address a range of topics including drug- and alcohol-related issues, alternatives to drug use (e.g. nutrition, training methods) and media/peer pressure resistance; and c) increase participant involvement and ownership in the programmes through peer-led teaching.[36]

The ninth finding notes the nascent but suggestive evidence linking PIEDS abuse with gateway, or facilitating, behaviours. Research in the context of adolescent and recreational sport suggests a relationship between a positive attitude toward doping or PIEDS use and the intention to use these substances.[37] Not surprisingly, individuals who have admitted to using illegal PIEDS have been found to have more positive attitudes to use than those who have not used them.[38] In addition, adolescent athletes' intention to use PIEDS is greater amongst those who perceive usage as meeting the approval of significant others (subjective norms), and are more convinced that the behaviour could be justified.[39] There is also evidence to suggest that PIEDS use intentions are influenced by the perceived prevalence of their use by other athletes (descriptive norms).[40] Furthermore, as we noted earlier, research demonstrates that those athletes who take nutritional supplements have more positive attitudes to doping and also hold a higher estimation of the use of performance enhancing substances.[41] One study found that dietary and nutritional supplement users were almost twice as likely to report use as compared to non-nutritional supplement users.[42] As this book, and others, have proposed, nutritional supplements may act as a 'gateway' to PIEDS use. However, it should be noted that attitudinal research around PIEDS has been criticised for its tendency to be descriptive and not always capable of establishing a causal relationship between attitudes and behaviour.[43] Additionally, it has been suggested that most previous research relies on under-developed theory and needs to better explore the complex social dynamics inherent with PIEDS use.[44]

Finally, the tenth finding in this analysis observes that while some supplements may work some of the time in some athletes,[45] there remains a great deal of confusion about the effects, veracity, risks and legality of different PIEDS. Towards this final problem, this primer provides a detailed PIEDS typology consisting of 15 types or categories.

Any attempt to typologise PIEDS is problematic due to the complexity of types, effects and compounds. For example, many different forms of PIEDS can be employed to target similar physical outcomes, but each may comprise a completely different composition, size of effect and risk profile. In order to account for the different nature of PIEDS, this primer classifies substances across three main strata, Dietary and Nutritional Supplements (DNS), Enhancement & Augmentation (EA) and Performance Enhancing Drugs (PEDS). For a simplified, 'snapshot' version of PIEDS based on effect type, size and risk, see Table 1.1.

Understanding PIEDS

Athletes at all levels, from community to elite sport, decide to use performance and image enhancing drugs and substances irrespective of the health, social and economic consequences.[46] Yet little empirical data exist explaining how decisions to use come about. For example, how do athletes go from using legal and relatively benign PIEDS like caffeine, codeine and curcumin to illegal or dangerous PIEDS like steroids, 'epo' (erythropoietin) and synthol? In this section, we compile the data in order to secure an improved, evidence-based understanding of PIEDS. It provides a classification of PIEDS types, physical impact, rates of use, user profiles and programme interventions.

PIEDS constitute any material an individual enters (through ingestion or injection) into, or applies on the surface of his or her body, to enhance physical performance or appearance. Included are pharmaceutical drugs (prescription, e.g. amphetamines; over-the-counter, e.g. alcohol, analgesics, caffeine; illicit, e.g. cocaine) and dietary or nutritional supplements (e.g. amino acids). Also included

TABLE 1.1 PIEDS by effects

Performance magnitude	Performance effect				
	Muscle Size Strength	Endurance Muscular Cardiovascular	Fat loss Stimulant Energy	Recovery Pain Inflammation Relaxation	Body appearance
LOW effect LOW risk	Testosterone boosters	(Most) Herbals	Aphrodisiacs fat burners (most)	(Most) Herbals	Fat-reducing applications
	Protein Amino acids Creatine monohydrate	Glucose electrolytes Beta-alanine HMB	Fat burners (e.g. CLA, Green tea, ACV)	Vitamins Minerals Glucose protein electrolytes Joint health (e.g. Glucosamine) Antioxidants (e.g. Fish oil, Curcumin, Vit. D, Resveratrol)	Sun tan sprays
			Calorie blockers	Sodium bicarbonate	
	Beta-2 agonists Exogenous AAS (e.g. Testosterone, Stanozolol, Nandrolone) Endogenous AAS (e.g. Androstenediol) SARMs	Beta-2 agonists	Energy drinks Caffeine Nitrates Nicotine Diuretics	Cough mixtures Antihistamines Alcohol Gluco-corticosteroids	Site enhancement (e.g. Silicone, Botox)
HIGH effect HIGH risk	Hormones (e.g. hGH, hCG, Somatropin, Insulin) Hormone antagonists & modulators (e.g. SERMs, Aromatase/ Myostatin Inhibitors)	Erythropoietin ACTH	Beta-2 agonists Ephedrine (and Pseudo-ephedrine) Amphetamines Adrenaline Cocaine	Beta-blockers Morphine Codeine Vicodin Cortisone Cannabinoids	Skin pigmentation (e.g. melatonin) Site enhancement (e.g. Synthol injections)

* Indicative examples used; not an exhaustive list of all PIEDS reviewed are substances athletes use for recreational, recovery or stress-management purposes, and which may be perceived as indirectly performance enhancing. PIEDS further encompass any substance used for augmenting aesthetic bodily appearance, but exclude cosmetics and 'cosmeceuticals' applied to the skin.

Despite the establishment of the World Anti-Doping Agency (WADA) in 1999, and the global spread of its 2003 Anti-Doping Code to ameliorate PIEDS use in elite sport, the problem of abuse and misuse remains complex and problematic, chiefly because the majority of use occurs at the non-elite, community level.[47] In fact, when PIEDS use includes dietary and herbal supplement consumption—including caffeine—the usage rates increase exponentially.[48] On the basis of a meta-analysis of available international studies, it has been estimated that more than 90% of all people who play sport, irrespective of performance level, have used some form of PIEDS to pursue a competitive benefit at some time in their sporting lives.[49]

The scope, magnitude and diversity of PIEDS use in sport and recreation make its study complex. A huge variety of PIEDS are available for athletes to apply, ingest or inject.[50] While a few substances such as alcohol, nicotine and caffeine have long been available, athletes can now employ a cocktail of stimulants, painkillers, anti-depressants, sedatives, muscle-building anabolic compounds, 'blood-boosting' hormones and illicit recreational drugs. Adding to these are ostensibly more benign DNS, ranging from mineral capsules, vitamin tablets, caffeinated energy drinks and carbohydrate bars to fatty acid compounds, protein supplements and plant extracts.

Although the dangers of some PIEDS use in sport are well rehearsed,[51] the majority of published studies have focused on clinical populations or case studies. These tend not to address the supra-therapeutic regimens and experimental combinations employed by athletes at all levels of performance, from the elite to the recreational.[52] The harms that can result from these practices are potentially severe and are often underestimated in the literature.[53] Some evidence even suggests that the most dangerous and prolific usage of PIEDS can be found in groups primarily interested in recreational performance and image enhancement, be it to build muscle, strip fat or iron-out cellulite.[54] Nevertheless, the use of PIEDS—and especially banned and illicit substances—has been linked to higher risks of depression, guilt and regret, lower self-esteem and negative body image.[55]

As noted earlier, the use of PIEDS to improve performance and appearance is related to an individual's drive to succeed, as well as the connection they feel between success and body perceptions. Data from Barkoukis et al., for example, predicted that any athlete who attributes his or her success to external factors would be more likely to use PIEDS in order to get ahead.[56] Just as many competitive athletes believe that success in elite sport cannot be achieved without PIEDS, so too do many recreational athletes think that their bodies require PIEDS in order to look better.[57] In a circuitous fashion, many elite athletes from a range of sports consider competitive success unlikely without PIEDS, while recreational trainers think that they can only look like competitive athletes by using PIEDS; they assume that PIEDS will compensate for a lack of genetic advantage, or that even the best athletes are using banned PIEDS.[58] Similarly, athletes at all levels harbour suspicions that dangerous PIEDS are significantly advantageous to not just sporting success, but to all the accoutrements that come with success in life generally, such as being physically attractive, peer admiration, perceptions of sexual prowess and economic gain.[59] Making the problem worse, 'defensive doping'—the practice of using banned or illicit PIEDS due to the belief that competitors are using them—may extend beyond elite sport as recreational trainers try to keep up with peers.[60] For example, adolescent non-competitive and recreational male users attempt to gain muscle size in order to bolster their physical appearance and sense of self worth within the context of their peers.[61] As a result, banned PIEDS use in sport and for improvements in physical appearance can become normalised.[62]

Elite athletes report that in order to reach the highest levels of performance it is necessary to go beyond naturally evolved talent by strategically employing PIEDS.[63] For example, elite cyclists have acknowledged that some serious substance use is needed to remain in the saddle.[64] Even those emerging elite athletes who claimed to avoid banned PIEDS reported that in order to achieve national or international success, additional banned PIEDS use would be essential.[65] For example, Lentillon-Kaestner and Carstairs[66] found that all of the young cyclists surveyed took some substances to improve their performances, and believed that it would not be possible to perform at that level without their use. Athletes from the lower levels of sport have indicated that in order to transition to the next level, some additional PIEDS use would be essential because at the professional and elite ranks, anything goes.[67]

Life courses

Recent evidence points to the critical relationship between athletes' PIEDS choices and their personal contexts, such as their physical and athletic career life cycles. Erickson et al.[68] duplicated a 2010 Australian study[69] on a smaller scale in the UK and reported that key transitions and instabilities during an athlete's life course increase their willingness to use heavier, often banned or illegal, PIEDS. Similarly, Hauw and McNamee's[70] data reinforced the pivotal relationships between athletes' PIEDS decisions and their career stages and circumstances.

Although Hauw and Bilard[71] predicted that athletes' PIEDS decisions follow a path connected to their sporting careers, athlete PIEDS decisions are likely to be far more dynamic and complex. In addition, PIEDS use may vary depending upon the level of performance, career stage and the nature of the sport's physical requirements. These variables imply that the content and timing of intervention policy will be most effective if targeted when athletes are at their most vulnerable to PIEDS abuse, or most open to change. This means that educational strategies must be available to athletes well before they face consequential decisions in the transition from community sport to more competitive levels. In addition, since

PIEDS use concentrates around community use, the need for education prior to the peer pressure and gender imaging of adolescence would seem critical.

Gateways to use

A few studies examining PIEDS use decisions have employed stepwise gateway and life-course theories. The so-called 'gateway' hypothesis—although controversial in mainstream substance use—holds that certain substances act as a gateway for the use of other substances, typically from those of lower risk to those of higher risk.[72] A growing body of research shows that as athletes advance along their life courses from recreational to elite performance—and from low body concern to high body concern—they also use more substances, newer substances and experimental combinations.[73]

By employing a linear sequence, gateway theory proposes that the use of lower-impact and lower-risk PIEDS might provide a facilitating pathway to the use of more impactful, higher-risk PIEDS.[74] As a result, the use of dietary supplements as a gateway to more powerful and possibly banned or illicit substances should be considered.[75] For example, numerous studies have established a relationship between the use of supplements and a later escalation towards banned and illicit PIEDS.[76] At least one study concluded that the supplements gateway increases the chances of later tobacco, alcohol or recreational drug use as well.[77]

Only a few studies have investigated whether gateway theory can provide a decisive explanation for athlete choices to use PIEDS. Backhouse et al.[78] determined that supplement users held more permissive attitudes to banned doping in sports than non-users. In addition, doping use was three and a half times more prevalent in supplement users compared to non-users. In general, supplement use correlates to more lenient attitudes towards sport doping in adolescents and athletes using legal PIEDS represent an at-risk group for the transition towards banned and illegal PIEDS.[79] Another study reported a relationship between the use of protein, creatine and anabolic steroids, where the use of each former substance provided a statistical predictor of the next.[80]

The nascent work in sport using life-course and gateway theories reveals some important pointers about PIEDS use. However, these theories remain linear and narrow and may miss significant variables affecting decisions to use. For example, Karazsia et al.'s[81] findings highlighted the need to connect sociocultural influences with gateway theory in order to explain decision making towards the use of riskier PIEDS. Other studies have highlighted that favourable views about PIEDS benefits can normalise their use.[82] They have also displayed the ways in which peer pressure in the form of social networks, external facilitators and inhibitors influences PIEDS use throughout an athlete's sporting life course.[83] In addition, the performance pathway for serious athletes may well differ from that of recreational athletes, especially since the latter are less concerned with whether a PIEDS is banned or not. The implication here is that, for the community user, fewer barriers preclude the transition from one level of PIEDS use to the next.

Although so-called gateway theories may deserve the critical scrutiny they have recently received in relation to recreational and illicit drugs,[84] our review of the sport and recreational context suggests that substance 'creep' should be taken seriously, especially when considered in light of emerging evidence connecting favourable perceptions of PIEDS benefits with use in elite sport.[85] In addition to more permissive attitudes[86] to banned or illegal PIEDS use by those using supplements, Barkoukis et al. concluded that the use of nutritional supplements is associated with biased reasoning in favour of doping.[87] In fact, young elite athletes who declare that supplementation is essential for sporting success are more likely to accept doping.[88]

Transitions between substances

Another important study indicated that body dissatisfaction, weight change behaviours and supplement use are related to more lenient attitudes towards sport doping in adolescents.[89] Even athletes from club-level sport who have rejected the use of banned substances seem to recognise that in order to effectively transition to the next level, some additional substance use remains essential.[90] Similarly, as we foreshadowed earlier, other research shows that while mid-level performing athletes fall short of using banned substances on a regular basis, they understand that in order to achieve national or international success, additional substance use is essential.[91] Furthermore, athletes' attitudes to banned substances are in part shaped by the attitudes and practices of fellow sport participants. Positive views about substance efficacy and appropriateness are likely to undermine effective regulation by normalising their use.[92]

In a mindset that so easily accommodates shifts in what constitutes dangerous PIEDS, many athletes experience substance use escalations over their competitive careers. Pain, sacrifice and psychological trauma are normal constituents in the athlete's routine; risk and health problems are part of the game. The threat of sanction, however severe, pales against a cost–benefit algorithm where failure is just as unpalatable as victory is compelling.[93] And that is before any economic incentives add impetus. To compound matters, elite athletes use prohibited PIEDS to bolster training and recovery more than to boost competition performances, leaving only out-of-season testing to sidestep. Studies have also revealed that it is possible for athletes to successfully use micro-dosing strategies in order to pass tests.[94] At the same time, community level athletes, and non-competitive trainers, remain at high risk of substance creep given the ready availability of the next substance, whether legal or not.

Conclusion

Athletes will experiment with almost any substance—banned or legal—if they believe it will improve their performances.[95] In one study it was revealed that subsequent to caffeine being removed from the WADA banned list, 74% of 20,686

Olympic athletes randomly tested for drug use had caffeine in their urine.[96] Many athletes place their performances over their health, while others have jettisoned any belief in immutable moral boundaries.[97] Our findings suggest that sport policy makers have a window of opportunity for guiding recreational and up-and-coming athletes into safe and legal PIEDS use through well-timed, evidence-based educational campaigns and regulatory pressures. Yet, we know little about why, how, and when athletes decide to use different PIEDS, including how information about such substances is sourced and evaluated, when athletes are most vulnerable or open to change, or the decision making that emerges as a consequence. While we pick up on some of these questions in later chapters, we first turn our attention to the widest end of the gateway funnel, dietary and nutritional supplements.

Notes

1 Honour, J. W. (2016). Doping in sport: Consequences for health, clinicians and laboratories. *Annals of Clinical Biochemistry: An International Journal of Biochemistry and Laboratory Medicine*, *53*(2), 189–190.
2 Kanayama, G., Pope Jr, H. G. & Hudson, J. I. (2001). "Body image" drugs: A growing psychosomatic problem. *Psychotherapy and Psychosomatics*, *70*(2), 61–65.
3 Pope Jr, H. G., Wood, R. I., Rogol, A., Nyberg, F., Bowers, L. & Bhasin, S. (2013). Adverse health consequences of performance-enhancing drugs: An Endocrine Society scientific statement. *Endocrine Reviews*, *35*(3), 341–375.
4 Iyer, R. & Handelsman, D. J. (2017). Testosterone Misuse and Abuse. In A. Hohl (ed.), *Testosterone* (pp. 375–402). Cham: Springer International Publishing.
5 Pope Jr, H. G., Wood, R. I., Rogol, A., Nyberg, F., Bowers, L. & Bhasin, S. (2013). Adverse health consequences of performance-enhancing drugs: An Endocrine Society scientific statement. *Endocrine Reviews*, *35*(3), 341–375.
6 Brennan, R., Wells, J. S. & Van Hout, M. C. (2016). The injecting use of image and performance-enhancing drugs (IPED) in the general population: A systematic review. *Health & Social Care in the Community*, 1–73.
7 Korkia, P. & Stimson, G. V. (1997). Indications of prevalence, practice and effects of anabolic steroid use in Great Britain. *International Journal of Sports Medicine*, *18*(7), 557–562.
8 Iversen, J., Topp, L., Wand, H. & Maher, L. (2012). Are people who inject performance and image-enhancing drugs an increasing population of Needle and Syringe Program attendees? *Drug Alcohol Review*, *32*, 205–207.
9 Gough, B., Seymour-Smith, S. & Matthews, C. R. (2016). Body dissatisfaction, appearance investment, and wellbeing: How older obese men orient to aesthetic health. *Psychology of Men & Masculinity*, *17*(1), 84–91.
10 Grogan, S. (2016). *Body Image: Understanding Body Dissatisfaction in Men, Women and Children*. London: Routledge.
11 Grogan, S. (2012). Body image development in adulthood. In T. F. Cash & L. Smolak (eds), *Body Image: A Handbook of Science, Practice, and Prevention* (pp. 93–100). New York: Guilford Press.
12 Gough, B., Seymour-Smith, S. & Matthews, C. R. (2016). Body dissatisfaction, appearance investment, and wellbeing: How older obese men orient to "aesthetic health". *Psychology of Men & Masculinity*, *17*(1), 84.
13 Brennan, R., Wells, J. S. & Van Hout, M. C. (2016). The injecting use of image and performance-enhancing drugs (IPED) in the general population: A systematic review. *Health & Social Care in the Community*, 1–73.

14 Ip, E. J., Barnett, M. J., Tenerowicz, M. J. & Perry, P. J. (2011). The Anabolic 500 survey: Characteristics of male users versus nonusers of anabolic-androgenic steroids for strength training. *Pharmacotherapy: The Journal of Human Pharmacology and Drug Therapy, 31*(8), 757–766.

15 Gonzalez, S. M. & Francis Keaney, A. (2001). Anabolic steroid misuse: How much should we know? *International Journal of Psychiatry in Clinical Practice, 5*(3), 159–167.

16 Brennan, R., Van Hout, M. C. & Wells, J. (2013). Heuristics of human enhancement risk: a little chemical help? *International Journal of Health Promotion and Education, 51*(4), 212–227.

17 Larance, B., Degenhardt, L., Copeland, J. & Dillon, P. (2008). Injecting risk behaviour and related harm among men who use performance-and image-enhancing drugs. *Drug and Alcohol Review, 27*(6), 679–686.

18 Smith, A. C. & Stewart, B. (2012). Body conceptions and virtual ethnopharmacology in an online bodybuilding community. *Performance Enhancement & Health, 1*(1), 35–38.

19 Brennan, B. P., Kanayama, G. & Pope, H. G. (2013). Performance-enhancing drugs on the Web: A growing public-health issue. *The American Journal on Addictions, 22*(2), 158–161.

20 Chandler, M. & McVeigh, J. (2014). Steroids and image enhancing drugs 2013 survey results. Liverpool, UK: LJMU Centre for Public Health.

21 Graham, M. R., Ryan, P., Baker, J. S., Davies, B., Thomas, N. E., Cooper, S. M., Evans, P., Easmon, S., Walker, C. J., Cowan, D. & Kicman, A. T. (2009). Counterfeiting in performance-and image-enhancing drugs. *Drug Testing and Analysis, 1*(3), 135–142.

22 Chandler, M. & McVeigh, J. (2014). Steroids and image enhancing drugs 2013 survey results. *Liverpool: LJMU Centre for Public Health*; Cooper, E. R., Kristine, C. Y. McGrath, X. L. & Heather, A. K. (2017). Androgen bioassay for the detection of non-labeled androgenic compounds in nutritional supplements. *International Journal of Sport Nutrition and Exercise Metabolism,* 1–26, doi.org/10.1123/ijsnem.2017-0018

23 Corazza, O., Bersani, F. S., Brunoro, R., Valeriani, G., Martinotti, G. & Schifano, F. (2014). The diffusion of performance and image-enhancing drugs (PIEDs) on the Internet: The abuse of the cognitive enhancer piracetam. *Substance Use & Misuse, 49*(14), 1849–1856.

24 Geyer, H., Parr, M. K., Koehler, K., Mareck, U., Schänzer, W. & Thevis, M. (2008). Nutritional supplements cross-contaminated and faked with doping substances. *Journal of Mass Spectrometry, 43*(7), 892–902.

25 Krug, O., Thomas, A., Walpurgis, K., Piper, T., Sigmund, G., Schänzer, W., Laussmann, T. & Thevis, M. (2014). Identification of black market products and potential doping agents in Germany 2010–2013. *European Journal of Clinical Pharmacology, 70*(11), 1303–1311.

26 Geyer, H. (2016). Adulterated nutritional supplements and unapproved pharmaceuticals as new sources of doping substances for fitness and recreational sports. *Doping and Public Health,* 31, 64–72.

27 Mottram, D. R., & Chester, N. (2014). Appendix: Synopsis of drugs used in sport. *Drugs in Sport, 326.*

28 Hatton, C. K., Green, G. A. & Ambrose, P. J. (2014). Performance-enhancing drugs: Understanding the risks. *Physical Medicine and Rehabilitation Clinics of North America, 25*(4), 897–913; Figueiredo, V. C. & Silva, P. R. P. D. (2014). Cosmetic doping— when anabolic-androgenic steroids are not enough. *Substance Use & Misuse, 49*(9), 1163–1167.

29 Brennan, R., Wells, J. G. & Van Hout, M. C. (2014). An unhealthy glow? A review of melanotan use and associated clinical outcomes. *Performance Enhancement & Health, 3*(2), 78–92.

30 Arent, S. M. & Lutz, R. S. (2015). The psychology of supplementation in sport and exercise: Motivational antecedents and biobehavioral outcomes. In M. Greenwood, D. S. Kalman & J. Antonio (eds), *Nutritional Supplements in Sports and Exercise* (pp. 23–48). London: Springer International Publishing.

31 Pope, H. G., Khalsa, J. H. & Bhasin, S. (2017). Body image disorders and abuse of anabolic-androgenic steroids among men. *JAMA*, *317*(1), 23–24.

32 Cafri, G., Olivardia, R. & Thompson, J. K. (2008). Symptom characteristics and psychiatric comorbidity among males with muscle dysmorphia. *Comprehensive Psychiatry*, *49*(4), 374–379; Olivardia, R., Pope Jr, H. G. & Hudson, J. I. (2000). Muscle dysmorphia in male weightlifters. A case-control study. *American Journal of Psychiatry*, *157*(8), 1291–1296; Phillips, K. A., Wilhelm, S., Koran, L. M., Didie, E. R., Fallon, B. A., Feusner, J. & Stein, D. J. (2010). Body dysmorphic disorder: Some key issues for DSM-V. *Depression and Anxiety*, *27*(6), 573–591.

33 Murray, S. B., Griffiths, S., Mond, J. M., Kean, J. & Blashill, A. J. (2016). Anabolic steroid use and body image psychopathology in men: Delineating between appearance- versus performance-driven motivations. *Drug and Alcohol Dependence*, *165*, 198–202.

34 Blouin, A. G. & Goldfield, G. S. (1995). Body image and steroid use in male bodybuilders. *International Journal of Eating Disorders*, *18*(2), 159–165.

35 Pereira, H. M. G. & Sardela, V. F. (2014). Stimulant doping agents used in Brazil: Prevalence, detectability, analytical implications, and challenges. *Substance Use & Misuse*, *49*(9), 1098–1114.

36 Backhouse, S. H., McKenna, J., Robinson, S. & Atkin, A. (2007). *Attitudes, Behaviors, Knowledge and Education—Drugs in Sport: Past, Present and Future.* Montreal, QC: World Anti-Doping Agency.

37 E.g., Lucidi, F., Zelli, A., Mallia, L., Grano, C., Russo, P. M. & Violani, C. (2008). The social–cognitive mechanisms regulating adolescents' use of doping substances. *Journal of Sports Sciences*, *26*(5), 447–456; Lucidi, F., Grano, C., Leone, L., Lombardo, C. & Pesce, C. (2004). Determinants of the intention to use doping substances, *International Journal of Sport Psychology*, *35*, 133–148; Zabala, M., Morente-Sanchez, J., Mateo-March, M. & Sanabria, D. (2016). Relationship between self-reported doping behavior and psychosocial factors in adult amateur cyclists. *The Sport Psychologist*, *30*, 68–75; Zelli, A., Mallia, L. & Lucidi, F. (2010). The contribution of interpersonal appraisals to a social-cognitive analysis of adolescents' doping use, *Psychology of Sport and Exercise*, *11*, 204–311.

38 Zabala, M., Morente-Sanchez, J., Mateo-March, M. & Sanabria, D. (2016). Relationship between self-reported doping behavior and psychosocial factors in adult amateur cyclists, *The Sport Psychologist*, *30*, 68–75.

39 Lucidi, F., Grano, C., Leone, L., Lombardo, C. & Pesce, C. (2004). Determinants of the intention to use doping substances. *International Journal of Sport Psychology*, *35*, 133–148; Zabala, M., Morente-Sanchez, J., Mateo-March, M. & Sanabria, D. (2016). Relationship between self-reported doping behavior and psychosocial factors in adult amateur cyclists, *The Sport Psychologist*, *30*, 68–75.

40 Lazuras, L., Barkoukis, V. & Tsorbatzoudis, H. (2015). Toward an integrative model of doping use: an empirical study with adolescent athletes. *Journal of Sport and Exercise Psychology*, *37*(1), 37–50.

41 Backhouse, S. H., Whitaker, L. & Petróczi, A. (2013). Gateway to doping? Supplement use in the context of preferred competitive situation, doping attitudes, beliefs and norms, *Scandinavian Journal of Medicine and Science in Sports*, *23*, 244–252; Barkoukis, V., Lazuras, L., Lucidi, F. & Tsorbatzoudis, H. (2015). Nutritional supplement and doping use in sport: possible underlying social cognitive processes. *Scandinavian Journal of Medicine & Science in Sports*, *25*(6), 1–7.

42 Barkoukis, V., Lazuras, L., Lucidi, F. & Tsorbatzoudis, H. (2015). Nutritional supplement and doping use in sport: possible underlying social cognitive processes. *Scandinavian Journal of Medicine & Science in Sports*, *25*(6), 1–7.

43 Backhouse, S., McKenna, J., Robinson, S. & Atkin, A. (2007). *Attitudes, Behaviours, Knowledge and Education—Drugs in Sport: Past, Present and Future.* Montreal, QC: World Anti-Doping Agency.

44 Backhouse, S., McKenna, J., Robinson, S. & Atkin, A. (2007). *Attitudes, Behaviours, Knowledge and Education—Drugs in Sport: Past, Present and Future*. Montreal: World Anti-Doping Agency.

45 Schwenk, T. L. & Costley, C. D. (2002). When food becomes a drug: Nonanabolic nutritional supplement use in athletes. *The American Journal of Sports Medicine*, *30*(6), 907–916.

46 Petróczi, A., Mazanov, J. & Naughton, D. P. (2011). Inside athletes' minds: Preliminary results from a pilot study on mental representation of doping and potential implications for anti-doping. *Substance Abuse Treatment, Prevention and Policy*, *6*(10), 1–8; Smith, A., Stewart, B., Oliver-Bennetts, S., McDonald, S., Ingerson, L., Anderson, A., Dickson, G., Emery, P. & Graetz, F. (2010). Contextual influences and athlete attitudes to drugs in sport. *Sport Management Review*, *13*(3), 181–197; Stewart, B. & Smith, A. (2010). Player and athlete attitudes to drugs in Australian sport: Implications for policy development. *International Journal of Sport Policy*, *2*(1), 65–84.

47 Stewart. B. & Smith A. (2014). *Rethinking Drug Use in Sport: Why the War will Never be Won*. London: Routledge; Turner, M. & McCrory, P. (2003). Social drug policies for sport: Athletes who test positive to social drugs should be managed differently from those who test positive for performance enhancing drugs. *British Journal of Sports Medicine*, *37*(5), 378–379.

48 Bojsen-Møller, J. & Christiansen, A. V. (2010). Use of performance and image-enhancing substances among recreational athletes: A quantitative analysis of inquiries submitted to the Danish anti-doping authorities. *Scandinavian Journal of Medicine & Science in Sports*, *20*(6), 861–867.

49 Stewart. B. & Smith A. (2014). *Rethinking Drug Use in Sport: Why the War will Never be Won*. London: Routledge.

50 Møller, V., Waddington, I. & Hoberman, J. M. (eds). (2015). *Routledge Handbook of Drugs and Sport*. London: Routledge.

51 Kaiser, B. & Smith, A. (2008). Globalization of anti-doping: The reverse side of the medal. *British Medical Journal*, 337, 85–87.

52 Evans-Brown, M., McVeigh, J., Perkins, C. and Bellis, M. (2012). *Human Enhancement Drugs: The Emerging Challenges to Public Health*. Liverpool, UK: JMU—Centre for Public Health.

53 Rahnema, C. D., Lipshultz, L. I., Crosnoe, L. E., Kovac, J. R. & Kim, E. D. (2014). Anabolic steroid-induced hypogonadism: Diagnosis and treatment. *Fertility and Sterility*, *101*(5), 1271–1279.

54 Evans-Brown, M., McVeigh, J., Perkins, C. & Bellis, M. (2012). *Human Enhancement Drugs: The Emerging Challenges to Public Health*. Liverpool, UK: JMU—Centre for Public Health.

55 Bloodworth, A. & McNamee, M. (2010). Clean Olympians? Doping and anti-doping: The views of talented young British athletes. *International Journal of Drug Policy*, *21*(4), 276–282; Lovstakken, K., Peterson, L. & Homer, A. L. (1999). Risk factors for anabolic steroid use in college students and the role of expectancy. *Addictive Behaviors*, *24*(3), 425–430.

56 Barkoukis, V., Lazuras, L. & Tsorbatzoudis, H. (2014). Beliefs about the causes of success in sports and susceptibility for doping use in adolescent athletes. *Journal of Sports Sciences*, *32*(3), 212–219.

57 Bloodworth, A. J., Petróczi, A., Bailey, R., Pearce, G. & McNamee, M. J. (2012). Doping and supplementation: The attitudes of talented young athletes. *Scandinavian Journal of Medicine & Science in Sports*, *22*(2), 293–301.

58 Calfee, R. & Fadale, P. (2006). Popular ergogenic drugs and supplements in young athletes. *Pediatrics*, *117*(3), e577–e589.

59 Lippi, G., Franchini, M., & Guidi, G. C. (2008). Doping in competition or doping in sport? *British Medical Bulletin*, *86*(1), 95–107; Moston, S., Engelberg, T. & Skinner, J. (2015). Self-fulfilling prophecy and the future of doping. *Psychology of Sport and Exercise*,

16, 201–207; Petroczi, A. & Strauss, B. (2015). Understanding the psychology behind performance-enhancement by doping. *Psychology of Sport and Exercise*, *16*, 137–139.

60/61 Bloodworth, A. J., Petróczi, A., Bailey, R., Pearce, G. & McNamee, M. J. (2012). Doping and supplementation: the attitudes of talented young athletes. *Scandinavian Journal of Medicine & Science in Sports*, *22*(2), 293–301.

62 Pappa, E. & Kennedy, E. (2013). "It was my thought . . . he made it a reality": Normalization and responsibility in athletes' accounts of performance-enhancing drug use. *International Review for the Sociology of Sport*, *48*(3), 277–294.

63 Cooper, C. (2012). *Run, Swim, Throw, Cheat: The Science Behind Drugs in Sport*. Oxford, UK: Oxford University Press.

64 Jeukendrup, A. & Tipton, K. D. (2009). Legal nutritional boosting for cycling. *Current Sports Medicine Reports*, *8*(4), 186–191; Jones, C. (2010). Doping in cycling: Realism, antirealism and ethical deliberation. *Journal of the Philosophy of Sport*, *37*(1), 88–101.

65 Stewart, B. & Smith, A. (2010). Player and athlete attitudes to drugs in Australian sport: Implications for policy development. *International Journal of Sport Policy*, *2*(1), 65–84.

66 Lentillon-Kaestner, V. & Carstairs, C. (2010). Doping use among young elite cyclists: a qualitative psychosociological approach. *Scandinavian Journal of Medicine & Science in Sports*, *20*(2), 336–345.

67 Lentillon-Kaestner, V. & Carstairs, C. (2010). Doping use among young elite cyclists: a qualitative psychosociological approach. *Scandinavian Journal of Medicine & Science in Sports*, *20*(2), 336–345.

68 Erickson, K., McKenna, J. & Backhouse, S. H. (2015). A qualitative analysis of the factors that protect athletes against doping in sport. *Psychology of Sport and Exercise*, *16*, 149–155.

69 Smith, A., Stewart, B., Oliver-Bennetts, S., McDonald, S., Ingerson, L., Anderson, A., Dickson, G., Emery, P. & Graetz, F. (2010). Contextual influences and athlete attitudes to drugs in sport. *Sport Management Review*, *13*(3), 181–197.

70 Hauw, D. & McNamee, M. (2015). A critical analysis of three psychological research programs of doping behaviour. *Psychology of Sport and Exercise*, *16*, 140–148.

71 Hauw, D. & Bilard, J. (2012). Situated activity analysis of elite track and field athletes' use of prohibited performance-enhancing substances. *Journal of Substance Use*, *17*(2), 183–197.

72 Kandel, D. B. (2002). *Stages and Pathways of Drug Involvement: Examining the Gateway Hypothesis*. Cambridge, UK: Cambridge University Press.

73 Petroczi, A. & Aidman, E. (2008). Psychological drivers in doping: The Life-cycle Model of performance enhancement. *Substance Abuse Treatment, Prevention, and Policy*, *3*(7), 3–12; Smith, A. & Stewart, B. (2012). Body perceptions and health behaviors in an online bodybuilding community. *Qualitative Health Research*, *22*(7) 971–985; Stewart, B. & Smith, A. (2010). Player and athlete attitudes to drugs in Australian sport: Implications for policy development. *International Journal of Sport Policy*, *2*(1), 65–84; Stewart, B. & Smith A. (2011). The role of ideology in shaping drug-use policies in Australian sport. *International Review for the Sociology of Sport*, *45*, 187–198; Stewart. B. & Smith A. (2014). *Rethinking Drug Use in Sport: Why the War will Never be Won*. London: Routledge.

74 Hildebrandt, T., Harty, S. & Langenbucher, J. W. (2012). Fitness supplements as a gateway substance for anabolic-androgenic steroid use. *Psychology of Addictive Behaviors*, *26*(4), 955–962; Yager, Z. & O'Dea, J. A. (2014). Relationships between body image, nutritional supplement use, and attitudes towards doping in sport among adolescent boys: implications for prevention programs. *Journal of the International Society of Sports Nutrition*, *11*, 13–21.

75 Metzl, J. D., Small, E., Levine, S. R. & Gershel, J. C. (2001). Creatine use among young athletes. *Pediatrics*, *108*(2), 421–425.

76 Backhouse, S. H., Whitaker, L. & Petróczi, A. (2013). Gateway to doping? Supplement use in the context of preferred competitive situations, doping attitude, beliefs, and norms. *Scandinavian Journal of Medicine & Science in Sports*, *23*(2), 244–252; Calfee, R. &

Fadale, P. (2006). Popular ergogenic drugs and supplements in young athletes. *Pediatrics*, *117*(3), e577–e589; Dodge, T. L. & Jaccard, J. J. (2006). The effect of high school sports participation on the use of performance-enhancing substances in young adulthood. *Journal of Adolescent Health*, *39*(3), 367–373; Lucidi, F., Zelli, A., Mallia, L., Grano, C., Russo, P. M. & Violani, C. (2008). The social–cognitive mechanisms regulating adolescents' use of doping substances. *Journal of Sports Sciences*, *26*(5), 447–456; Papadopoulos, F. C., Skalkidis, I., Parkkari, J. & Petridou, E. (2006). Doping use among tertiary education students in six developed countries. *European Journal of Epidemiology*, *21*(4), 307–313.

77 Yussman, S. M., Wilson, K. M. & Klein, J. D. (2006). Herbal products and their association with substance use in adolescents. *Journal of Adolescent Health*, *38*(4), 395–400.

78 Backhouse, S. H., Whitaker, L., & Petróczi, A. (2013). Gateway to doping? Supplement use in the context of preferred competitive situations, doping attitude, beliefs, and norms. *Scandinavian Journal of Medicine & Science in Sports*, *23*(2), 244–252.

79 Yager, Z. & O'Dea, J. A. (2014). Relationships between body image, nutritional supplement use, and attitudes towards doping in sport among adolescent boys: implications for prevention programs. *Journal of the International Society of Sports Nutrition*, *11*, 13–21.

80 Karazsia, B. T., Crowther, J. H. & Galioto, R. (2013). Undergraduate men's use of performance-and appearance-enhancing substances: An examination of the gateway hypothesis. *Psychology of Men & Masculinity*, *14*(2), 129–137.

81 Karazsia, B. T., Crowther, J. H. & Galioto, R. (2013). Undergraduate men's use of performance- and appearance-enhancing substances: An examination of the gateway hypothesis. *Psychology of Men & Masculinity*, *14*(2), 129–137.

82 Petróczi, A. (2007). Attitudes and doping: A structural equation analysis of the relationship between athletes' attitudes, sport orientation and doping behaviour. *Substance Abuse Treatment, Prevention, and Policy*, *2*(1), 34–49; Petróczi, A., Mazanov, J. & Naughton, D. P. (2011). Inside athletes' minds: Preliminary results from a pilot study on mental representation of doping and potential implications for anti-doping. *Substance Abuse Treatment, Prevention and Policy*, *6*(10), 1–8.

83 Petroczi, A. & Aidman, E. (2008). Psychological drivers in doping: The Life-cycle Model of performance enhancement. *Substance Abuse Treatment, Prevention, and Policy*, *3*(7), 3–12.

84 Bell, K. & Keane, H. (2014). All gates lead to smoking: The "gateway theory", e-cigarettes and the remaking of nicotine. *Social Science & Medicine*, *119*, 45–52; Kleinig, J. (2015). Ready for retirement: The gateway drug hypothesis. *Substance Use & Misuse*, *50*(8–9), 1–5.

85 Petróczi, A. & Aidman, E. (2008). Psychological drivers in doping: The Life-cycle Model of performance enhancement. *Substance Abuse Treatment, Prevention, and Policy*, *3*(7), 3–12; Petróczi, A., Mazanov, J. & Naughton, D. P. (2011). Inside athletes' minds: Preliminary results from a pilot study on mental representation of doping and potential implications for anti-doping. *Substance Abuse Treatment, Prevention and Policy*, *6*(10), 1–8.

86 Backhouse, S. H., Whitaker, L. & Petróczi, A. (2013). Gateway to doping? Supplement use in the context of preferred competitive situations, doping attitude, beliefs, and norms. *Scandinavian Journal of Medicine & Science in Sports*, *23*(2), 244–252.

87 Barkoukis, V., Lazuras, L., Lucidi, F. & Tsorbatzoudis, H. (2015). Nutritional supplement and doping use in sport: possible underlying social cognitive processes. *Scandinavian Journal of Medicine & Science in Sports*, *25*(6), 1–7.

88 Bloodworth, A. J., Petroczi, A., Bailey, R., Pearce, G. & McNamee, M. J. (2012). Doping and supplementation: The attitudes of talented young athletes. *Scandinavian Journal of Medicine & Science in Sports*, *22*(2), 293–301.

89 Yager, Z. & O'Dea, J. A. (2014). Relationships between body image, nutritional supplement use, and attitudes towards doping in sport among adolescent boys: Implications for prevention programs. *Journal of the International Society of Sports Nutrition*, *11*, 1–8.

90 Lentillon-Kaestner, V. & Carstairs, C. (2010). Doping use among young elite cyclists: A qualitative psychosociological approach. *Scandinavian Journal of Medicine & Science in Sports, 20,* 336–345.

91 Smith, A., Stewart, B., Oliver-Bennetts, S., McDonald, S., Ingerson, L., Anderson, A., Dickson, G., Emery, P. & Graetz, F. (2010). Contextual influences and athlete attitudes to drugs in sport. *Sport Management Review, 13*(3), 181–197.

92 Petroczi, A. & Aidman, E. (2008). Psychological drivers in doping: The life-cycle model of performance enhancement. *Substance Abuse Treatment, Prevention, and Policy, 3,* 3–12; Petróczi, A., Mazanov, J. & Naughton, D. P. (2011). Inside athletes' minds: Preliminary results from a pi lot study on mental representation of doping and potential implications for anti-doping. *Substance Abuse Treatment, Prevention and Policy, 6,* 1–8.

93 Lippi, G., Franchini, M. & Guidi, G. C. (2008). Doping in competition or doping in sport? *British Medical Bulletin, 86*(1), 1–10.

94 Ashenden, M., Gough, C. E., Garnham, A., Gore, C. J. & Sharpe, K. (2011). Current markers of the Athlete Blood Passport do not flag microdose EPO doping. *European Journal of Applied Physiology, 111*(9), 2307–2314.

95 Smith, A., Stewart, B., Oliver-Bennetts, S., McDonald, S., Ingerson, L., Anderson, A., Dickson, G., Emery, P. & Graetz, F. (2010). Contextual influences and athlete attitudes to drugs in sport. *Sport Management Review, 13*(3), 181–197; Wiefferink, C. H., Detmar, S. B., Coumans, B. Vogels, T. & Paulussen, T. G. (2008). Social psychological determinants of the use of performance-enhancing drugs by gym users. *Health Education Research, 23*(1), 70–80.

96 Del Coso, J., Muñoz, G. & Muñoz-Guerra, J. (2011). Prevalence of caffeine use in elite athletes following its removal from the World Anti-Doping Agency list of banned substances. *Applied Physiology, Nutrition, and Metabolism, 36*(4), 555–561.

97 Hamilton, T. & Coyle, D. (2013). *The Secret Race: Inside the Hidden World of the Tour de France: Doping, Cover-ups, and Winning at all Costs.* London: Random House.

2

POWER, PLEASURE, FAT AND FIT

Dietary and nutritional supplements as PIEDS

Introduction

Dietary and nutritional supplements (DNS) use has become a taken-for-granted practice in modern society. DNS cover a wide variety of substances, and range from concentrated mineral capsules, vitamin tablets and carbohydrate bars to fatty acid compounds, protein drinks and plant extracts.[1] There is little regulation over DNS use, and, as a result, the claims that are made for their health- and fitness-giving properties are frequently extravagant, and often short on evidence. Despite the problematic status of many DNS, their use has exploded over recent times and there are many people who testify to their capacity to aid healing, reduce pain, increase energy levels, improve physical appearance, speed up recovery and, more generally, increase longevity.

DNS occupy a pivotal place in the health product sector, and involve significant levels of consumer spending. Over the past two decades especially, their use has exploded. In the largest market, the US consumption of DNS more than doubled between 1990 and 1997, when it increased from $US6.5 billion to just under $US13 billion.[2] By 2010 total DNS sales were valued at $US20 billion[3] and are estimated to climb above $US30 billion within a few years. Projections place the global market at $US278 billion by 2024.[4]

Due to escalating interest in Western methods of weight loss and health amongst Japan, China and India, DNS sales in the broader Asia region have become the largest geographical growth centre, accounting for almost half of global revenue. In addition, the proliferation of e-commerce portals, including AliBaba and Made-In-China, is anticipated to drive demand to dizzying heights in the forthcoming decade. Connected to this development, the Australian market is enjoying growth of around 6% a year given its Asia Pacific export focus. In fact, according to recent Roy Morgan research, the Chinese market has an insatiable appetite for Australian-made DNS.[5] Domestic interest also seems to be increasing, with between eight and nine million (approximately 45% of the population) Australians purchasing DNS every year totalling around $AUS1 billion. Approximately one-third of the revenue comes from exports.[6]

When compared to the last available data from the Australian Bureau of Statistics compiled in 2011–2012, the escalation in use appears dramatic, from around 25% of the population just five years ago to nearly half today.[7] Although the US, European and Chinese markets dwarf Australian revenues, Australians are actually the largest users of DNS on a per capita basis in the world.

Despite market variations, in general, the largest-selling DNS items are vitamins, consumed predominantly by women between 35 and 64 years of age. Men under 25 are the least interested in vitamins, but are the most interested in sports supplements. From a growth perspective, however, no DNS enjoys the current popularity of protein bars.

What are dietary and nutritional supplements?

There has been a problem in defining the term 'dietary and nutritional supplements', and part of the reason for this is the lack of agreement on just what range of substances the term is supposed to cover, and what words best capture the functions they are supposed to perform. They have been labelled as nutritional supplements, multi-nutritional preparations, nutritional ergogenic aids and sports supplements.[8]

According to one authority, DNS can be best described as a three-pronged class of substances that covers: 1) multi-vitamins and multi-minerals; 2) amino acids of various types; and 3) various herbs and exotic plants that go under the general heading of botanicals.[9] According to the US Food and Drug Administration, a DNS is a product—excluding tobacco—that is intended to supplement the diet and bears or contains one or more of the following dietary ingredients: a vitamin, a mineral, a herb or other botanical, an amino acid, a dietary supplement for use by humans to supplement the diet by increasing its total daily intake, or a concentrate, a metabolite, constituent, extract or combination of these ingredients.[10]

Supplements abound for every stage in a consumer's activity routine, typically structured around at least five specific times: 1) pre-exercise (e.g. stimulants/energy drinks, fat-burners, fatigue delayers, energy/fuel suppliers, muscle-builders); 2) during exercise (energy/fuel suppliers, fatigue delayers); 3) post-exercise (e.g. recovery boosters, muscle synthesisers, energy and electrolyte replacers); 4) meal time (e.g. calorie-blockers, health supporters, anti-inflammatories); and 5) prior to sleep (e.g. muscle-synthesisers, anti-oxidants, sleep aids, health supporters).[11] In addition, some supplements—especially those linked to image enhancement—may be consumed or used either habitually (e.g. fat-burners, calorie-blockers) or at irregular intervals (e.g. botulinum toxin—e.g. Botox, aphrodisiacs, tanning substances).

DNS are often viewed as attractive options to banned or illegal PIEDS for a growing number of athletes at all levels. There are a number of reasons for this.

First, they are not illegal; second, they are easily sourced; third, they are relatively benign; and fourth, they can still improve performance, if only at the margin in some instances. So, at first glance, there seems to be little to worry about when it comes to DNS use. Their very name implies a capacity to improve well-being in the most natural of ways, and they are seen to be a convenient way to top up one's food intake and to make sure that all the essential vitamins, minerals, carbohydrates, proteins and trace elements are supplied to the body in the right amounts. And, unlike most of the illicit drugs that are pushed onto the black market, they do not appear to lead to serious illness, physical dependency or addiction.

However, a number of concerns accompany the use of DNS. First, they are not tested for safety and efficacy in the same ways as prescription and other pharmaceutical drugs. Second, their distribution is poorly regulated. Third, users are often poorly informed, and badly advised about the benefits they might expect to secure from the supplements. As our review foreshadows, most supplements have little to no performance impact to speak of, and are therefore little more than hideously expensive placebos. In other words, many DNS are effectively a waste of money, and there is little evidence to confirm that they improve performance in any significant way. Fourth, a worrying volume of evidence suggests that imported DNS may be subject to contamination, or contain ingredients not identified by the label. For example, methylhexaneamine (also known as DMAA), an illegal substance with dangerous side effects, has been found in supplements and has been linked to a death in Australia. Finally, there is the possibility of serious health risks associated with heavy dosages and experimental combinations, and these risks are often poorly communicated to athletes.

Patterns of DNS use

The use of DNS to improve performance has increased rapidly over recent years. Anywhere between 44%[12] and 100%[13] of elite athletes use DNS, with the usage rate depending on age, sport and level of competition. A study of sport practices in Finland found that 66% of track and field athletes used at least one supplement.[14] Another Finnish study found an even higher level of use amongst elite athletes. Heikkinen et al.,[15] when looking at the 2002 Olympic Games athlete cohort, found that 81% had used dietary supplements. In a follow-up analysis in 2009, the number of dietary supplement users had fallen to 73%. Multi-vitamin preparations were the most frequently cited, with 54% using them in 2002 and 57% using them in 2009. The two other most popular products were protein powders (47% and 38%) and vitamin C (28% and 24%), respectively. The heaviest users were the 24+ years age group. It was also found that males used more dietary supplements than females, and that endurance athletes had a much higher usage rate than those who played a team sport of one sort or another. On the other hand, athletes in speed and power events had higher usage rates than team sport participants.

In a Canadian study of elite athletes, just over 88% took at least one DNS on a regular basis.[16] The most frequently declared dietary supplements were sport drinks at 22%, sports bars at 14%, multivitamin and minerals at 13%, protein supplements at 9% and finally, vitamin C at 6%. In a study of the American population between 2003 and 2006, 49% had used some form of DNS, with female use (53%) slightly higher than male use (44%). Multi-vitamins and multi-minerals were used most frequently (33%), followed by botanical supplements (14%) and amino acids (4%). For adults, the use level was 54%, while for people over 70 years of age the use level was an age-cohort high of 70%.[17] Older studies of German and New Zealand adult residents show a daily usage rate of 35–45%.[18]

In an Australian study of elite swimmers preparing for the 2000 Sydney Olympic Games, 94% had taken some type of non-food supplements. The most popular supplements were multi-vitamin or multi-mineral supplements, which were used by every supplement user. Sports drinks—being heavily spiked with caffeine, carbohydrates and herbal preparations—and creatine monohydrate—a high-energy phosphate that turbo-charges the body's muscular contraction systems—were the next most popular supplements. Their usage levels were 87%, 61% and 31%, respectively.[19] A study of Sri Lankan athletes found an even higher dietary supplement usage rate. Overall, just over 94% said they had recently used some form of supplement.[20]

The most recent meta-analysis reported that elite athletes used DNS far more than recreational athletes. In addition, usage was similar for men and women with the exceptions that more women used iron, while more men used vitamin E, creatine and protein.[21]

Motives for use

The factors that motivate DNS use amongst athletes are multi-fold. Most of the data indicate that athletes take supplements in order to maintain sound levels of health, sustain intensive training regimes, improve physical appearance—including the addition of lean body mass at the same time as reducing body fat—and secure a competitive edge in either or both sporting events and peer esteem. In a Finnish study, athletes used supplements to support recovery from training and optimise performance.[22] In a Canadian study, 32% of respondents indicated they used DNS to increase energy.[23] The other main drivers of use in this study were the desire to maintain health, at 27%, the need to better recover from exercise, at 19%, and the aim of enhancing immunity, at 14%. In a Sri Lankan study, 79% of all informants said they took DNS to enhance performance, while 20% consumed supplements to improve their general health status. The most popular products were multi-vitamin preparations (with a usage rate of 80%), calcium supplements (54%), vitamin E (52%), energy foods (45%), creatine (40%) and electrolyte-replacement drinks (38%). Slightly more exotic products like branch-chain amino acids and herbal-sourced stimulant preparations had a use level of under 5%.[24] The heaviest users were older track and field athletes, while the lightest users were younger footballers.

Influences on use

DNS are often viewed as an attractive option to banned substances, since they are legal, easily sourced, have no serious negative side effects, and improve performance, if only a little. While some players and athletes use their own research to work out what might be a suitable compound to ingest, others look for guidance. The intent to use certain supplements by adolescents—as well as their attitudes towards them—is affected by pivotal social influencers surrounding them such as peers, coaches and parents.[25] Widespread use and communication about supplements can be normalised as a result. In addition, athletes at all levels receive often conflicting information about the risks associated with the use of various DNS from agenda-driven and unreliable sources like the Internet, fellow competitors, magazines, friends, amateur coaches, supplement labels, retail sales staff and, worst of all, supplement marketing.[26] The best-informed individuals have only fragments of scientific data to consult about the possible risks of DNS,[27] a consequence of the vast number on the market, often short product life cycles, constant new offerings with ever greater claims, and the resource and time intensity needed to conduct efficacious research.[28]

In a study of Australian swimmers, 53% reported that they valued the advice of dieticians, doctors, pharmacists and sport scientists most highly. The opinions of coaches were also sought out, but they were considerably lower on the DNS-advice pecking order, with only 30% of informants rating coach views as essential inputs. The least credible sources of advice were seen to be alternative nutritional practitioners such as health food shop sales assistants, herbalists and naturopaths, with less than 10% of informants ranking them in their top three sources of advice. Testimonials from other players and athletes were also given a low ranking, although their views were rated more highly than 'alternative' nutritional practitioners.[29] The results from a study of Sri Lankan athletes were similar, with 45% of informants rating sport doctors as the most important source of advice. The next most highly rated sources were team coaches and friends, at 40% and 15%, respectively.[30]

Concerns about use

At first glance, there seems to be little to worry about when it comes to DNS use. Their very name implies a capacity to simply and conveniently improve well-being naturally. In other words, they are perceived as a benign way to top up one's food intake, and to make sure that all the essential vitamins, minerals, carbohydrates, proteins and trace elements are supplied to the body in the right amounts. And, it is typically assumed that, unlike most of the illicit drugs that are pushed onto the black market, they do not lead to serious illness, physical dependency or addiction.

Yet, there are a number of concerns that come with the use of freely available DNS. Of uppermost concern is the fact that DNS are not tested for safety and efficacy in the ways that prescription and other pharmaceutical drugs are. There is no requirement that DNS be clinically tested and trialled before approval by governments before being distributed for sale. At the moment there are few controls, even in developed nations, apart from the common legislated consumer protection requirement that there will be no misleading advertising or unsubstantiated claims about a product's efficacy. Other than a handful of stalwart supplements, the majority have received little or no empirical attention.[31]

There are potential health risks associated with heavy dosages of DNS, and these risks are often poorly communicated to users. In fact, some medical authorities claim that a high level of DNS use in sport situations is not defensible on medical grounds.[32] In short, they cause mild to moderate levels of harm when overused. Even the most commonly used supplements have predominantly been studied under short-term clinical conditions. Long-terms effects—and side effects—remain unclear.[33] At the same time, the misuse of ostensibly benign supplements such as protein powders can lead to health disturbances including stress on major organs.[34] Far more alarming is the potential for low-risk and even health-supporting supplements to become contaminated[35] by toxic or high allergenic ingredients[36] in the absence of independent manufacturing quality controls and the virtually unrestricted importation of unregulated products. Further studies have demonstrated that labelling accuracy poses a severe problem,[37] in some cases revealing a difference of 15–20% between ingredient terminologies and their actual presence.[38] A recent review found a disturbing 'adulteration' of dietary supplements by the illegal introduction of synthetic drugs.[39]

In addition, users are often poorly informed and ill-advised about the benefits they might expect to secure from supplements. As we will explore later, the weight of evidence suggests that most DNS have a marginal performance impact. A good portion of DNS is effectively a waste of money, and there is little evidence that confirms that they improve performance in any significant way.

Conclusion

Overall, there is a high degree of ambiguity and ambivalence around DNS use in every level of sport. No one knows how prevalent DNS use is beyond the most rudimentary estimates based on market sales, and similarly little is known about which DNS are most popular, and why. No data on frequency and dosages are available at all. Furthermore, it remains unclear what sporting practices involve more or less supplement use than others, or the extent to which usage occurs completely outside of sport performance objectives. There are few data to tell us what users think they actually get from their DNS use. And, neither do any empirical data inform us what either stops users from moving into the banned and illegal substances on the one hand, or 'incentivises' them to step up to the 'harder' performance enhancing drugs (PEDS) on the other. Neither can we say whether DNS use is linked to prescription drug use, nor under what conditions the two are mutually supportable. Finally, we can only speculate on what ethical position users take on the consumption of DNS. There remains a dearth of research material in and around DNS use that can inform sport authorities and policy makers on how best to reduce the physical and social risks that accompany escalating use. In the following chapter we expand our analysis leading to an evaluation of the scale and scope of all PIEDS use.

Notes

1 Williams, M. H. (2015). Dietary supplements for endurance athletes. In E. S. Rawson & S. L. Volpe (eds), *Nutrition for Elite Athletes* (pp. 45–63). Boca Raton, FL: CRC Press.
2 Baylis, A., Cameron-Smith, D. & Burke, L. (2001). Inadvertent doping through supplement use by athletes: Assessment and management of the risk in Australia. *International Journal of Sport Nutrition and Exercise Metabolism, 11*, 365–383.
3 Skolnik, H. & Chernus, A. (2010). *Nutrient Timing for Peak Performance*. Champaign, IL: Human Kinetics.
4 Grand View Research, Inc. (2016). *Global Dietary Supplements Market*, San Francisco, CA: Grand View Research.
5 Roy Morgan Single Source (Australia), July 2014–June 2015.
6 RSM International Limited (2016). Industry snapshot: Vitamin and supplement manufacturing. A snapshot of the key statistics and current industry performance in the vitamin and supplement manufacturing sector. London: RSM International Limited.
7 Australian Bureau of Statistics (2011–2012). Australian health survey: Nutrition first results—Foods and nutrients, 2011–2012, 4364.0.55.007.
8 Braun, H., Koehler, K., Kleinert, J., Mester, J. & Schanzer, W. (2009). Dietary supplement use amongst elite young German athletes. *International Journal of Sport Nutrition and Exercise Metabolism, 19*, 97–109; Smith, C., Wilson, N. & Parnell, W. (2005). Dietary supplements: Characteristics of supplement users in New Zealand. *Nutrition and Dietetics, 62*(4), 123–129.
9 Bailey, R. L., Gahche, J. J., Lentino, C. V., Dwyer, J. T., Engel, J. S., Thomas, P. R., Betz, J. M., Sempos, C. T. & Picciano, M. F., 2010. Dietary supplement use in the United States, 2003–2006. *The Journal of Nutrition*, jn-110.
10 Braun, H., Koehler, K., Kleinert, J., Mester, J. & Schanzer, W. (2009). Dietary supplement use amongst elite young German athletes. *International Journal of Sport Nutrition and Exercise Metabolism, 19*, 97–109; Housman, J., Dorman, S., Pruitt, B., Ranjita, M. & Perko, M. (2011). Consumption of sport-related dietary supplements among NCAA Division 1 female student athletes. *American Journal of Health Behavior, 35*(4), 438–446.
11 Naderi, A., de Oliviera, E. P., Ziegenfuss, T. N. & Willems, M. E. (2016). Timing, optimal dose and intake duration of dietary supplements with evidence-based uses in sports nutrition. *Journal of Exercise Nutrition & Biochemistry*, eprints.chi.ac.uk/id/eprint/1989.
12 Braun, H., Koehler, K., Kleinert, J., Mester, J. & Schanzer, W. (2009). Dietary supplement use amongst elite young German athletes. *International Journal of Sport Nutrition and Exercise Metabolism, 19*, 97–109.
13 Housman, J., Dorman, S., Pruitt, B., Ranjita, M. & Perko, M. (2011). Consumption of sport-related dietary supplements among NCAA Division 1 female student athletes. *American Journal of Health Behavior, 35*(4), 438–446.
14 Tscholl, P., Alonso, J., Dolle, G., JUnge, A. & Dvorak, J. (2010). The use of drugs and nutritional supplements in top-level track and field athletics. *American Journal of Sports Medicine, 38*(1), 133–140.
15 Heikkinen, A., Aleranta, A., Helenius, I. & Vasankari, T. (2011). Use of dietary supplements in Olympic athletes is decreasing: A follow up study between 2002 and 2009. *Journal of the International Society of Sports Nutrition, 8*(1), 1–8.

16 Erdman, K. A., Fung, T. S., Doyle-Baker, P. K., Verhoef, M. J. & Reimer, R. A. (2007). Dietary supplementation of high-performance Canadian athletes by age and gender. *Clinical Journal of Sport Medicine*, *17*(6), 458–464.

17 Bailey, R. L., Gahche, J. J., Lentino, C. V., Dwyer, J. T., Engel, J. S., Thomas, P. R., Betz, J. M., Sempos, C. T. & Picciano, M. F. (2010). Dietary supplement use in the United States, 2003–2006. *The Journal of Nutrition*, ju-110.

18 Reinert, A., Rohrmann, S., Becker, N. & Linseisen, J. (2007). Lifestyle and diet in people using dietary supplements. *European Journal of Nutrition*, *46*(3), 165–173; Smith, C., Wilson, N. & Parnell, W. (2005). Dietary supplements: Characteristics of supplement users in New Zealand. *Nutrition and Dietetics*, *62*(4), 123–129.

19 Baylis, A., Cameron-Smith, D. & Burke, L. M. (2001). Inadvertent doping through supplement use by athletes: assessment and management of the risk in Australia. *International Journal of Sport Nutrition and Exercise Metabolism*, *11*(3), 365–383.

20 de Silva, A., Samarasinghe, Y., Senanayake, D. & Lanerolle, P. (2010). Dietary supplement intake in national-level Sri Lankan athletes. *International Journal of Sport Nutrition and Exercise Metabolism*, *20*(1), 15–20.

21 Knapik, J. J., Steelman, R. A., Hoedebecke, S. S., Austin, K. G., Farina, E. K. & Lieberman, H. R. (2016). Prevalence of dietary supplement use by athletes: Systematic review and meta-analysis. *Sports Medicine*, *46*(1), 103–123.

22 Tscholl, P., Alonso, J. M., Dollé, G., Junge, A. & Dvorak, J. (2010). The use of drugs and nutritional supplements in top-level track and field athletes. *The American Journal of Sports Medicine*, *38*(1), 133–140.

23 Erdman, K. A., Fung, T. S., Doyle-Baker, P. K., Verhoef, M. J. & Reimer, R. A. (2007). Dietary supplementation of high-performance Canadian athletes by age and gender. *Clinical Journal of Sport Medicine*, *17*(6), 458–464.

24 de Silva, A., Samarasinghe, Y., Senanayake, D. & Lanerolle, P. (2010). Dietary supplement intake in national-level Sri Lankan athletes. *International Journal of Sport Nutrition and Exercise Metabolism*, *20*(1), 15–20.

25 McNamee, M. (2009). Beyond consent? Paternalism and pediatric doping. *Journal of the Philosophy of Sport*, *36*(2), 111–126.

26 Herriman, M., Fletcher, L., Tchaconas, A., Adesman, A. & Milanaik, R. (2017). Dietary supplements and young teens: Misinformation and access provided by retailers. *Pediatrics*, e20161257; Welthagen, A. (2016). The development of a measuring instrument to determine the knowledge and attitudes of elite adolescent athletes about ergogenic aids and banned substances (Doctoral dissertation, University of the Free State).

27 Despite the problematic information reliability issues that the Internet presents, it has also facilitated the emergence of numerous resources a vigilant coach or athlete could consult. For example, ConsumerLab.com provides independent testing and reviews of thousands of dietary supplements, specified by brand names. The database is available for a site licence fee. The site has received external validation (see Hogan Smith, K. (2017). Review of ConsumerLab. com: A database of dietary supplements. *Journal of Consumer Health on the Internet*, *21*(1), 95–102.

28 Morente-Sánchez, J. & Zabala, M. (2013). Doping in sport: A review of elite athletes' attitudes, beliefs, and knowledge. *Sports Medicine*, *43*(6), 395–411.

29 Baylis, A., Cameron-Smith, D. & Burke, L. M. (2001). Inadvertent doping through supplement use by athletes: assessment and management of the risk in Australia. *International Journal of Sport Nutrition and Exercise Metabolism*, *11*(3), 365–383.

30 de Silva, A., Samarasinghe, Y., Senanayake, D. & Lanerolle, P. (2010). Dietary supplement intake in national-level Sri Lankan athletes. *International Journal of Sport Nutrition and Exercise Metabolism*, *20*(1), 15–20.

31 Cohen, P., Geller, A., Budnitz, D., Eichner, A., Travis, J. & Venhuis, B. (2016). Safety of dietary supplements. *Planta Medica*, *82*(05), OA47; Sirota, L. (2015). Dietary supplements: Safety, efficacy and quality. *Journal of Nutrition Education and Behavior*, *47*(5), 485-e1.

32 Tscholl, P., Alonso, J. M., Dollé, G., Junge, A. & Dvorak, J. (2010). The use of drugs and nutritional supplements in top-level track and field athletes. *The American Journal of Sports Medicine*, *38*(1), 133–140.

33 Baume, N., Hellemans, L. & Saugy, M. (2007). Guide to over-the-counter sports supplements for athletes: Review article. *International SportMed Journal*, *8*(1), 2–10; Deldicque, L. & Francaux, M. (2016). Potential harmful effects of dietary supplements in sports medicine. *Current Opinion in Clinical Nutrition & Metabolic Care*, *19*(6), 439–445.

34 Nieper, A. (2005). Nutritional supplement practices in UK junior national track and field athletes. *British Journal of Sports Medicine*, *39*(9), 645–649.

35 Cohen, P. A., Travis, J. C. & Venhuis, B. J. (2015). A synthetic stimulant never tested in humans, 1, 3-dimethylbutylamine (DMBA), is identified in multiple dietary supplements. *Drug Testing and Analysis*, *7*(1), 83–87.

36 Geyer, H., Parr, M. K., Koehler, K., Mareck, U., Schänzer, W. & Thevis, M. (2008). Nutritional supplements cross-contaminated and faked with doping substances. *Journal of Mass Spectrometry*, *43*(7), 892–902.

37 Berginc, K. & Kreft, S. (eds). (2014). *Dietary Supplements: Safety, Efficacy and Quality*. London: Elsevier.

38 Wang, Y., Adam, T. J. & Zhang, R. (2016). Term coverage of dietary supplements ingredients in product labels. In *AMIA Annual Symposium Proceedings*, *2016*, 2053. American Medical Informatics Association.

39 Rocha, T., Amaral, J. S. & Oliveira, M. B. P. (2016). Adulteration of dietary supplements by the illegal addition of synthetic drugs: A review. *Comprehensive Reviews in Food Science and Food Safety*, *15*(1), 43–62.

3

USE, ABUSE, PATTERNS AND PROFILES

Scale and scope of PIEDS use in sport

Introduction

Over the last 50 years there have been growing concerns about the increasing amount of drug and substance use in sport and recreation at all levels. Today, drug use constitutes a multi-dimensional problem that begins with everyday substances like alcohol and caffeine, moves into over-the-counter drugs that contain stimulants or analgesics, goes into prescription drug use that involves even heavier stimulant and analgesic effects, shifts into performance enhancement drugs, and finishes up with potent recreational drugs. Some of these substances deliver marked improvements to athletic performances (and body composition), which most sporting officials judge to be intolerable since it creates a tilted playing field where already well-resourced players and athletes obtain an even greater advantage through access to new products as they become available.[1]

Drug use is thus viewed as a corrupt practice that undermines the integrity of sporting contests, and should be seen as analogous to the moral bankruptcy displayed in match fixing.[2] Within such a social context, it came as no surprise that a global anti-doping regime arose in the form of the World Anti-Doping Agency (WADA). This all happened in 1999, and it was anticipated that WADA's presence—and especially its punitive powers—would clean up the drug use problem within a decade. However, nearly two decades later it remains unclear as to whether the WADA-driven anti-drug stance has reduced either the incidence or prevalence of drug use in sport. In fact, a good case can be made for the claim that use has actually increased.[3] Certainly, WADA's presence has done nothing to restrain the enthusiastic uptake of substances for image enhancing purposes.

When it comes to understanding the scale and scope of the PIEDS use problem in sport and recreation, five questions immediately come to mind: first, what types of drugs and related substances are being used? second, who takes them? third, how frequently are they used? fourth, what is the intent behind their use? and, finally, where does use take place?

In order to answer these questions, we dig deeply into a broad array of empirical studies, government reports, sport industry surveys, drug testing results, drug agency investigations, scholarly commentaries, the writings of journalists and the revelations of users. But, getting a clear picture of the extent of PIEDS use around sport and the community is not as simple as it seems. This is, in part, the result of disagreement about just what constitutes PIEDS and 'drugs' in particular, and which drugs can demonstrably improve performance or body composition.[4] The sport and public policy waters are further muddied by disputes over how illicit drugs should be treated, the legitimacy of prescription drug use and exactly where supplements fit.[5] Despite these challenges, we located sufficient data to establish a suggestive picture of the scale and scope of drug use in sport. Unfortunately, our conclusions about PIEDS use in sport and the community suffer from an absence of objective research evidence. Our discussion begins with the prevalence of use.

Prevalence of drug use in sport and the community

The use of PIEDS is endemic in elite sport, but they are also employed in non-sporting contexts by individuals seeking to improve their appearance, mostly through a combination of muscle gain and fat loss. The focus of the general news media is on the professional athletes who are caught using hormonal drugs, most commonly, AAS. However, the majority of individuals using PIEDS are recreational athletes who use them to improve overall strength and personal appearance.[6] Conclusive evidence demonstrates that the use of substances such as AAS, growth hormone, erythropoietin and stimulants poses significant health risks including cardiovascular disease, diabetes, cancer, mental health issues, virilisation in females and the suppression of naturally produced androgens in males.[7]

In one survey of 500 AAS users, nearly four out of five were non-athletes with cosmetic objectives. AAS users in this sample were taking larger doses than ever previously recorded; more than half of the respondents were using a weekly AAS dose in excess of 1000 mg, which is 10–20 times more than the average male body manufactures naturally per week. The majority of these steroid users self-administered AAS by intramuscular injection, and approximately one in 10 users reported hazardous injection techniques. Poly-pharmacy was practised by more than 95% of AAS users, with one in four users taking growth hormone and insulin. Nearly 100% of AAS users reported subjective side effects.[8] Serious body-builders and other athletes used insulin, especially in concert with other hormones like human growth hormone, with which synergistic effects were elicited. For example, one web-based survey identified 41 non-diabetic insulin users, of whom 95% also used AAS and practised poly-pharmacy.[9]

Reported rates of PEDS use amongst elite athletes ranged between 5% and 31%, depending upon the survey. The most commonly used PEDS were AAS, human growth hormone, erythropoietin (and blood doping), amphetamines and stimulants.[10] A meta-analysis reported that the global lifetime prevalence rate of AAS was 3.3%. The prevalence rate for males, 6.4%, was significantly higher than the rate for females, 1.6%.[11] According to other recent studies, the prevalence of AAS dependence among AAS users has been estimated to be approximately 30%, with poly-substance use including growth hormone and insulin-like growth factor.[12]

Few studies examining the knowledge bases of PIEDS users return encouraging results. In Iran, for example, one study concluded that most football coaches and players had a poor or moderate understanding of prohibited drugs and their side effects.[13] Worse, they seemed to hold a range of factually incorrect assumptions and colloquial myths about PIEDS.

Anecdotal accounts of use

A common view amongst officials, politicians and commentators holds that sport throughout the world faces a PIEDS use epidemic. Many high-profile international incidents have reinforced this claim, with the 2016 exposé of embedded drug use in Russia's track and field programme being a recent case.[14] Professional road cycling has also received significant attention, featuring allegations of doping connected to its most famous event, the Tour de France.[15] It culminated in the highly-publicised investigation of Lance Armstrong, who was found to have used banned performance enhancing substances for much of his professional cycling career. In addition, track and field athletes have yielded numerous high-profile positive tests, the most explosive incident involving Marion Jones who, along with several other prominent athletes, became embroiled in the BALCO scandal.[16] These incidents created enormous angst amongst sport's stakeholders. But, as Lentillon-Kaestner and Ohl have argued,[17] the selective use of cases places some uncertainty over the prevalence of drug use in sport, exactly what type of drugs are being used and what performance or personal gains they are expected to deliver.

Be that as it may, from an anecdotal viewpoint, and as reported in the media, a drug scourge in sport has not only tilted the playing field in favour of those players with close pharmaceutical connections, but has also destroyed sport's capacity to bolster the moral fibre of its participants. Media reports often trade on 'moral panic' by connecting drug use in sport with social chaos. In these instances, colourfully exaggerated stories are dredged up from the past leading to calls for restoring control through some top-down regulatory mechanism, typically involving coercion, fines, suspensions and even jail sentences.

A classic case of moral panic arose out of a US Judiciary hearing into steroid use in 1989, when Pat Connolly, a coach of the women's track and field team, claimed that 15 out of the 50-strong women's team at the 1984 Los Angeles Olympics had used steroids on a regular basis. Moreover, she noted that some of them were medallists.[18] Connolly elaborated that drug use escalated even further for the 1988 Seoul Olympics, estimating that at least 40% of the women's team had likely used steroids at some time during their Games preparation.[19]

In Australia, in 2002, a serious case of moral panic similarly erupted when an Australian rules footballer suggested that 80% of elite players had some experience with recreational drugs.[20] This created enormous consternation amongst the football community,[21] and the only consolation the media could offer officials and fans were quotes from other players who said the figure was nearer 30%.[22] While mainstream media-driven narratives tend to have an element of truth in them, they also revel in juicy scandals and as a result need to be tempered by a broader base of evidence through first, athlete drug-testing data, and second, studies that have secured information about athletes' attitudes and behaviours regarding drug use. As with all research, we should lend most weight to results guided by sound protocols and trusted methodologies.

Results of drug-testing regimes

We begin our survey of the scale and scope of banned drug use around the world by reviewing the data compiled by the International Olympic Committee (IOC) and WADA over recent years. These figures reveal that throughout the 1990s less than 2% of all drug test results were positive, exhibiting inappropriate levels of banned substances. The most commonly used drugs were AAS—or what we frequently refer to as 'steroids'—which accounted for 1131 positive tests in 1996, 856 tests in 1998, 946 in 2000, 1191 in 2004, 3259 in 2008 and 3400 in 2012. The 2012 figure accounted for 55% of all positive tests. The next most frequently used drugs were beta-agonists, more commonly known as the active ingredients in various forms of anti-asthma and respiratory management medications. They accounted for 350 positive tests in 2008. Stimulants also seem to be substances of choice, accounting for 281 positive tests in 1996, 412 in 1998, 453 in 2000, 382 in 2004 and 472 in 2008. At the same time, peptide hormones (which include erythropoietin [EPO]), delivered fewer positive tests, with four in 1996, 12 in 1998, 12 in 2000, 78 in 2004 and 106 in 2008. Although cannabis and its derivatives are not, technically speaking, performance enhancing drugs, they remain banned during competition. For both 2004 and 2012 there were more positive tests for so called 'cannabinoids' (518 and 560, respectively) than there were for stimulants (382 and 502).

At the 2000 Sydney Olympic Games just over 2800 tests were conducted, including 310 tests for EPO. However, these tests yielded only 12 positive results (five of which involved steroids), amounting to just 0.47% of all tests. Similarly, the positive test figures for the 2002 Salt Lake City Winter Games were modest. Only five of 1960 tests were positive, not even 0.3% of all tests. At Athens, in 2004, 26 athletes tested positive to banned substances, but when taken in the context of nearly 3700 tests, they accounted for only 0.7%. Torino in 2006, and Beijing in 2008, delivered even lower positive test rates. Nearly 4800 drug tests were undertaken at Beijing, but only 0.42% delivered a positive result, which was slightly lower than Sydney.[23]

The low positive test rates for the Olympics need to be tempered by the results of studies undertaken in the broader sporting community. Independent studies of elite athletes by sport scientists in Norway[24] and the UK[25] each found a banned drug usage rate of less than 2%. These are slightly higher than the IOC/ WADA drug test figures, but hardly suggest an epidemic of illegal drug use running rampant through the global elite sporting community.

By most standards, the positive test rates during the 1990s and into the 2000s seem pleasingly low. Equally, most sport commentators have conceded that the officially measured rates underestimated the true level of banned drug use.[26] There are three reasons for this. First, most drug use occurs during periods of intense training rather than in competition, but for many years most testing was done excusively in periods of competition. Second, some drugs were not detectable and therefore did not show positive in any tests. Third, athletes utilise masking agents and methods—other legal drugs, compounds and techniques that camouflage the presence of banned substances in their systems. As a result of these three challenges to accurate testing, researchers employ surveys of athletes and players in the hopes of securing a more plausible picture of drug use in sport.

Surveys of reported drug use

Numerous surveys have sought to establish realistic levels of drug use in sport, as well as the ethical attitudes players and athletes hold towards use. The surveys have focused on both the broad community and sport participants, utilising a range of techniques such as questionnaires and in-depth interviews. Results indicate a complex range of reported usage levels of banned substances, with varying usage levels for different drug types and sport practices.

Community surveys

During the late 1980s and 1990s, a series of revealing studies examined anabolic steroid usage. According to a study of high school male adolescents in the US, around 11% were current or previous anabolic steroid users.[27] This figure was, however, treated with caution when other studies found that only 2.5% of adolescent males used steroids. Subsequent studies found a 5% usage rate amongst young men aged 18, with a 3% rate for those participating in sporting competitions.[28] One broad-ranging study reported caffeine as the drug of choice, given the 27% of all informants declaring that they used it regularly. Alcohol and painkillers came in at around 9%, while stimulants generated a usage level of just 3%.[29]

Parkinson and Evans undertook another revealing community study of drug use.[30] Having noted that less than 3% of young American adults had taken steroids at least once in their lives, the researchers invited 500 anabolic steroid users to complete a web-based questionnaire. The results revealed that just under 80% had used steroids for what they called 'cosmetic reasons', which meant they were mainly concerned with looking good and feeling strong. Dosage levels also varied enormously between respondents, with 40% not going beyond 1000 mg per week, but 26% regularly exceeding 1500 mg on a weekly basis. Additionally, just under 25% reported that they practiced poly-pharmacy, which meant in this case that they complemented their steroid use with growth hormone and/or insulin. While 60% of respondents said they were concerned about the possible negative side effects—with acne, testicular shrinkage, insomnia, sexual dysfunction, injection site pain, fluid retention and mood changes front and centre—only 37% had discussed their steroid use with a physician. Finally, the respondents admitted to securing their steroids mainly from illegal sources, with 50% obtaining their supplies from 'bootleg' operators and illicit laboratories.

A Finnish study of nearly 11,000 male conscripts with an average age of 19 years also provided some illuminating results. Matilla et al.[31] asked these young men to comment on their substance use and health status. Some of the questions invited participants to record their use of anabolic steroids, and if they did initially use, to explain what provided them with the incentive to continue. It was found that only 0.9% of respondents had used anabolic steroids over their lifetime, a figure well below those from other studies. According to Matilla's team, American studies had shown a usage rate of 3–11% while European studies had shown prevalence rates of 2–3%.

What caused such low levels of anabolic steroid usage amongst this cohort of 19-year-old Finnish conscripts was unclear. It was noted, however, that high use levels had been previously associated with engagement in weight-training programmes at fitness centres, frequent drunkenness, daily smoking and low levels of educational attainment. Similarly, a Jordanian survey of gym users reported that 8.2% of the sample regularly used medication for performance or image purposes without a prescription. Usage was equally divided by gender. Various forms of testosterone, hormones and fat burners (stimulants and beta-2 agonists) were the most popular substances.[32]

The claim that gyms and fitness centres can be the catalyst for an increase in steroid use was supported by Striegel's research. This 2006 study invited around 620 members of fitness centres in Germany to complete a survey about gym practices and substance use.[33] Just under 14% of respondents had used steroids at some point during their fitness centre activities. When asked to identify their motives for using, more than 80% of respondents emphasised the importance of building a better-looking and stronger body, while only 8% were interested in improving their levels of fitness and sporting performances. In addition, around 30% of users employed additional substances to enhance the bodily impact. Clenbuterol (designed to treat breathing disorders like asthma, but also effective in raising the body's metabolic rate and reducing body fat) and stimulants like ephedrine were recorded as the most popular 'add-ons'. When users were asked to identify the source of their training 'products', just over half cited the 'black market'. In practice, this meant acquiring supplies from friends and informal contacts. Fewer than 50% of users had also accessed pharmacies for some of their complementary products as well.

Player and athlete surveys

Player and athlete surveys provide a different perspective on drug and related substance use. One of the earliest but most extensive studies of players and athletes was undertaken in 1991, and delivered the startling finding that 64% of informants believed that at least one of their fellow athletes used drugs on a regular basis.[34] Similarly, Pearson and Hanson completed a survey of US Olympic athletes around the same time, and found that many athletes had either used or knew of others who used.[35] Just under 44% of those who completed the survey believed that at least one in 10 of their peers were taking some sort of performance enhancing substance, while another 34% estimated that somewhere between 1% and 9% of their colleagues were using. In subsequent studies of endurance athletes, 41% of informants thought that some of their team-mates were taking performance enhancing drugs.[36]

In 1998, the *Independent* newspaper in the UK surveyed 300 elite players and athletes, reporting that more than 50% considered sport to be contaminated with drug use.[37] Responses varied between sport categories, with the highest response rate coming from weightlifters, where every one of them thought drug use permeated their sport. When questioned about their own drug use, just over 40% of the 300 elite players and athletes admitted to using caffeine in order to secure a competitive edge, 15% admitted to using testosterone, 15% admitted to using some form of stimulant while 8% admitted to using narcotic analgesics.

A study of 706 English professional footballers confirmed the problematic and pervasive nature of drug use in sport.[38] Of all respondents surveyed, 34% claimed that other players were commonly using performance enhancing drugs (PEDS) although only 6% indicated a personal knowledge of PEDS-taking players. Interestingly, only 29% of informants suggested that other players were taking recreational drugs, although when questioned about personally knowing someone who took them, 45% responded positively.

In a 2006 study by Alaranta et al., 44% of power sport participants declared that they personally knew of other athletes who used banned substances, while 37% of endurance athletes harboured similar suspicions.[39] The argument for thinking that positive drug test ratios consistently underestimate 'real' drug use levels was further supported by a study done by Uvacsek et al. completed in 2009. In this study, 82 Hungarian athletes were invited to talk about their drug use attitudes and behaviours. The results revealed that around 15% of all respondents admitted to using performance enhancing substances, about 32% admitted to using recreational and/or illicit drugs.[40] It was also found that users overestimated the drug use of others when compared to non-users. For example, where those who doped imagined that on average 35% of others doped, non-dopers provided an average estimate of 17%. In the case of recreational drug use, users anticipated that 51% of all others used, while for the non-users, the figure was a much lower 39%.

Another revealing study was undertaken by Dunn et al., who used a web-based survey of 214 Australian exercising males who had not previously used anabolic steroids, to obtain a better understanding of what so-called 'rank and file' participants do to improve their physical appearances and general levels of well-being.[41] It was initially found that 80% of all respondents used some form of supplement or conditioning aid to assist them in their 'body improvement' projects. Illicit substance use was also common, with 52% of respondents admitting to administering amphetamines, cannabis, inhalants, cocaine, off-label narcotic analgesics or sedatives in the previous six months. There were no reports of heroin use. At the same time, when asked to comment on their views about anabolic steroids, 16% said they were likely to use some form of synthetic testosterone in the future as a way of getting stronger and more muscular.

There is now a significant amount of data showing that substance use amongst elite athletes is more common than was initially anticipated. For example, in 2014 Mosten et al. found that 21% of 92 coaches believed that the use of PEDS was common amongst most sports, with 31% believing that cycling was the most problematic.[42] Kissalita and Robinson, in a 2014 study of American sportspeople, found that 8% of competitive cyclists used banned PEDS while 60% used PIEDS that were not banned.[43] In a similar vein, a 2011 study of Indian athletes by Neeraj et al. found that 22% had used banned substances at some time during their careers.[44]

In recent times two additional revelations have confirmed that the use of banned substances can sometimes be orchestrated by a coterie of administrators, coaches and sport scientists on an organised basis. In the 2013–2016 Essendon Football Club case, the Australian Court of Arbitration for Sport found that 34 players had consented to injections of a banned peptide hormone,[45] while the entire Russian track and field team were banned from competing at the Rio de Janeiro Games on the grounds that they had comprehensively failed to comply with the WADA drug use controls, used PIEDS on a regular basis and sabotaged drug-testing processes with scant regard for the principles of transparency and fair play.[46] In 2017, the entire winter Olympics team from the Russian Federation was banned from competing under their country's flag in the 2018 PyeongChang Games.

It should come as no surprise to discover that sport participants, especially at the highly competitive level, would not only contemplate use but also go the whole distance. At the very least they would think about using performance enhancing substances. On the other hand, it is often argued that sport participation can act as a shield against recreational drug use, since it ingrains the idea that sport can only be played properly if its participants have a clear head and a well-functioning body. With this logic, we would anticipate that people who play more sport would use fewer recreational drugs. However, the data suggest that sport participation does not necessarily discourage recreational drug use.

During the 2008–2009 period, two research teams—Peck et al.[47] and Wichstrom and Wichstrom[48]—found that adolescent participation in team sports, especially those rewarding aggression, often led to an increase in alcohol and cannabis use in early adulthood. Peck et al. reported that adolescents who both played sports and were already consuming moderate levels of alcohol were highly susceptible to heavy drinking in early adulthood. Another—albeit earlier—study of university athletes determined that 96% of informants drank alcohol regularly, with just over 20% smoking cannabis and 18% popping painkillers.[49]

When it comes to elite sport, the relationship between drugs and lifestyle becomes even more perplexing. Peretti-Watel et al. surveyed 460 elite student athletes in France, concluding that the overall prevalence of cigarette, alcohol and cannabis use was less than half the rate of non-athlete students.[50] However, girls competing at an international level were more likely to smoke cigarettes and cannabis, perhaps due to the belief that their consumption would alleviate competitive stress and anxiety. Finally, the study revealed that adolescent athletes involved in team sports were more prone to drink alcohol at least once a month.

While providing some revealing insights about drug use in sport, including the probability that it is widespread and multifaceted, the survey results we have summarised also raise some additional questions. For example, overall do players and athletes actually use drugs more often than non-players and athletes? Surveys of university athletes point to some answers.

Surveys of students

At first glance, it would seem reasonable to think that university students, especially those who regularly play sport, would be cautious about drug use, whether performance enhancing or recreational. Furthermore, as these students suffer from time pressures, it would also be reasonable to think that they cannot afford to undermine the capacities of their bodies and minds to work hard and long. In fact, the opposite appears to be the case. For example, North American college students describe alarmingly high rates of drug use. In one study, about 70% of college students admitted to drinking alcohol at least once in the month before the survey, while 40% reported intermittent binge drinking. In another study of US college students, about 18% used illicit drugs during the 12 months prior to the survey.[51]

The trend persists through further studies of college athletes, who have higher rates of substance use than college non-athletes, and generally engage in more high-risk behaviours.[52] Alcohol presents the case in point. For example, Ford's 2007 study of US colleges concluded that college athletes used alcohol more freely than non-athletes.[53] Where 49% of male non-athletes engaged in binge-drinking, the number increased to 54% for athletes. Similarly, 29% of female non-athletes claimed to binge-drink while the figure for athletes climbed to 39%. On the other hand, male athletes had lower cannabis and illicit drug use, of 26% and 12%, respectively, compared to 31% and 16% for non-athletes. The general theme of these findings was reinforced by results from Eitle et al. in their 2003 study of American high schools, which found that playing high school sport was positively associated with alcohol use.

Some evidence also reveals that different substance usage rates apply to different sports. For example, in Ford's study,[54] while 75% of male college ice hockey players indulged in binge-drinking, the percentage decreased to around 41% for track athletes and runners. Reported cannabis use also varied between sports, with a usage rate of 39% for male ice hockey players but only 19% for basketballers. Differences emerged for females as well, with 47% of soccer players binge drinking compared with only 27% of runners. Based on the available evidence, drug usage varies considerably depending on the substance type and sporting code. When it comes to the use of anabolic steroids and synthetic testosterone, the usage rate among university student athletes was normally less than 10%, but was also three times higher when bodybuilders were involved.[55] For example, the Tahtamouni et al. 2008 study of Jordan University student athletes and bodybuilders found that 4% of athletes used banned AAS, while 26% of bodybuilders used AAS.[56] The results for US studies of university students are similar. Dodge et al.'s. 2014 study of US college athletes found that while just under 1% had used AAS, a much higher 8% had used prescription stimulants without approval.[57] Karazsia et al., in their 2013 study, found that 6% of US college athletes took illegal substances and that 96% of this 6% reported earlier protein use, while 85% reported creatine use, both of which are legal.[58] These results predict that a gateway model was at work, whereby the less powerful but permissible substances were stepping-stones to more esoteric and dangerous PIEDS use.

Australian studies of young people in a sporting context also depict a relatively high use of drugs and related substances. An alarming level of alcohol consumption has been especially evident. In a 2004 study, Duff et al.[59] discovered that 88% of community sport club members regularly drank alcohol on club premises. Of that 88%, around 23% drank at their club on at least two occasions per week. Another 41% said they drank alcohol at the club on average once per week. When asked to explain the cultural factors influencing the pattern of drinking at their club, just over 80% of respondents agreed with the statement that 'drinking is a good way to relax after training or after playing a match', 79% agreed that 'drinking is an important part of club camaraderie', while 77% agreed with the statement that 'drinking is an important part of celebrating' after the game.

While teenage athletes had lower usage rates than university athletes, they were nevertheless exposed to the seductive qualities of PEDS and banned substances. A 1999 study of an American high school football team by Stilger and Yesalis provided a sharp insight into drug use in local community settings.[60] The researchers initially found that around 6% of team members had used anabolic steroids. When asked to explain their use, 47% said they did it to improve their athletic performance, 29% did it to improve their appearance and 14% said they did it to keep up with the competition. When asked to respond to the statement, 'I would use anabolic-androgenic steroids if I knew opponents playing against me were using it', 54% of the players who had used confessed that they would do it again. Those students who had previously used also said they had no difficulty securing their steroids, with 30% getting them from athletes outside of school, 29% getting them from team-mates and friends, 25% getting them from a local doctor and 19% obtaining their supplies from their school coach.

In 2011, Dunn and White found that 2.4% of Australian teenagers had used AAS on a regular basis.[61] The figures for US teenage high school students were even higher. Rees et al. found that 8% of high school students used AAS regularly, while 22% used protein supplements on a steady basis.[62] Eisenber et al. found that 6% of high school boys and 5% of girls had used AAS at least once in the previous 12 months. Protein powder use was 35% and 23%, respectively.[63] In 2010, Goulet et al. found that 25% of junior Canadian athletes—a surprisingly high figure—had used illegal substances to improve performance.[64]

In Iceland, a 2011 study by Thorlindsson and Halldorsson returned a teenage student usage rate of just under 2%,[65] while a 2014 study by Nolte et al. into South African junior athletes found that 4% had used banned substances.[66] Furthermore, 14% said they would consider using if they had little chance of being found out. In Europe, Wanjek et al. found that 15% of German high school students had used at least one substance on the WADA banned list during the previous 12 months.[67] However, these substances were, for the most part, not performance enhancing. The most frequently used substance was cannabis, while under 1% of the students surveyed used AAS.

A recent US-based survey of college students showed that individuals who had participated in at least one sport during high school had a greater chance of an on-and-off opioid medical prescription for their lifetimes, compared with non-active respondents.[68] Usage of opioid painkillers climbs with the seriousness of the user. For example, in the US, NCAA level college athletes use serious painkillers regularly[69] while NFL players use them all the time.[70] In fact, opioid use amongst NFL players has been described in epidemic terms.[71] Image users may not be far behind, with bodybuilders, powerlifters, weightlifters[72] and gym junkies all regular consumers.[73] Studies suggest that AAS use may lead to an imbalance in the neurotransmitter systems governing the biochemical reward process, creating a greater sensitivity toward opioid narcotics and stimulants.[74]

Overall, there is an expectation that many athletes will use some type of performance enhancing substance, and it has become a fact of life for most sport participants. The results of a 2015 study by Morenta-Sanchez and Zebela encapsulates the ways in which PIEDS have become ingrained in so many sporting leagues and cultures.[75] The study surveyed 273 coaches, trainers and technical staff, including doctors, sport scientists and physiotherapists. Every participant cohort had an experience involving the use of PIEDS. Around 35% knew of athletes who were using banned substances, while 16% knew of athletes who had incited others to use.

In-depth qualitative research using player and athlete interviews

Although now dated, Anshel undertook one of the more illuminating qualitative drug investigations in sport studies in 1991. It provided a detailed analysis of: 1) player attitudes to drug use; 2) the reported and perceived incidence of drug use in elite-level sport; and 3) the motives for using different types of drugs.[76] Anshel conducted a series of in-depth interviews with 126 elite American athletes, comprising 94 males and 32 females, over a 3-year period beginning in 1986. The results showed that 64% of all informants were aware of some type of illegal drug use in their sports. The figures were higher for male athletes (72%) than for female athletes (40%). When questioned about performance enhancing drug use, 64% of informants responded positively while a marginally smaller 63% indicated that some of their colleagues and team-mates were taking a form of illicit recreational drug. The most commonly used drugs were perceived to be anabolic steroids, amphetamines, diuretics, painkillers and narcotic analgesics, cannabis, hallucinogens and anti-depressants.

When informants were asked to explain what motivated them to take drugs, they referred primarily to the need to be competitive, such as becoming stronger and faster. The next frequently cited motivators included the desire to better cope with stress, the desire for fun, satisfying curiosity about the effects of different drugs, the importance of being able to better manage pain and the need to avoid failure. Some significant gender differences were linked with these motivators. For example, where 29% of male informants cited the need to increase energy and help 'psyche-up' as a prime motivator, the equivalent for females was only 1%. The responses were reversed when it came to resolving personal problems as a motivator, with just over 32% of females citing it compared with only 1% of males.

Conclusion

Despite the shortage of studies examining drug use in general amongst sporting populations, a few insightful studies have focused on steroid use in the broader community. For example, Petrocelli et al. undertook one such study in 2008, which involved a series of semi-structured interviews with 37 steroid users who frequented gyms in various US states.[77] The researchers began their study by noting the problems anabolic steroids can generate. A number of earlier studies suggested that unsupervised steroid use, especially amongst teenagers, was associated with poor self-esteem, elevated rates of depression, a greater risk of attempting suicide, little knowledge of positive health issues, concerns about body weight, eating disorders, increased rates of violent behaviour and an unhealthy obsession with being strong and building muscle.

The material reviewed in this chapter confirms that people who combined gym work with steroid use were doing it to build a stronger and more muscled body. It was also evident that nearly every one of the respondents felt the need to use steroids because their aspirations for a heavily muscled body were unlikely to be attained under a standard gym work routine. These 'frustrations' led the informants to seek out substances that would enable them to 'get huge' and 'get ripped'. Similarly, most respondents declared that steroid use not only helped them build muscle, but also made them feel more confident and, surprisingly, often calmer and more rational, thus offsetting the claim that steroid use was unavoidably linked to 'roid rage'. The steroid users had, for the most part, a strong inner feeling of raw, primitive strength and enthusiasm.

Neither were the informants overly concerned about the risks steroid use posed to their long-term health. When asked to comment on side effects such as hair loss, infertility, aggression and liver damage, respondents tended to critique these claims as unbelievable, and even intentionally manipulative on the part of the medical community and government. Instead, the major concerns voiced were first, the high financial costs of maintaining their training and supplementation regimes, and second, the problems they encountered with doctors when aiming to secure their supplies legally. For the older users, doctors had to be convinced that the request for synthetic testosterone and human growth hormone was important to restoring testosterone levels back to those associated with fit and active young men. What remains now is the question of to what extent cultural and contextual factors affect PIEDS use.

Notes

1 Bloodworth, A. & McNamee, M. (2010). Clean Olympians? Doping and anti-doping: The views of talented young British athletes. *International Journal of Drug Policy*, *21*(4), 276–282; Dunn, M., Thomas, J. O., Swift, W., Burns, L. & Mattick, R. P. (2010). Drug testing in sport: The attitudes and experiences of elite athletes. *International Journal of Drug Policy*, *21*(4), 330–332; Henne, K. (2010). WADA, the promises of law and the landscapes of antidoping regulation. *PoLAR: Political and Legal Anthropology Review*, *33*(2), 306–325.

2 Bricknell, S. (2015). Corruption in Australian sport. *Trends and Issues in Crime and Criminal Justice*, *490*, 1.

3 See, for example, Sean Ingles, Russia faces complete ban from 2018 Winter Paralympics over doping scandal. *The Guardian*, 22 May 2017. Sourced from www.theguardian.com/sport/2017/may/22/russia-ban-2018-winter-olympics-doping-scandal

4 Backhouse, S., McKenna, J., Robinson, S. & Atkin, A. (2007). Attitudes, behaviours, knowledge and education. *Drugs in Sport: Past, Present and Future*. Montreal: World Anti-Doping Agency.

5 Breivik, G., Hanstad, D. V. & Loland, S. (2009). Attitudes towards use of performance-enhancing substances and body modification techniques. A comparison between elite athletes and the general population. *Sport in Society*, *12*(6), 737–754.

6 O'Hagan, A. & Walton, H. (2015). Bigger, faster, stronger! An overview of anabolic androgenic steroids and their use and impact on the sport industry. *Forensic Research & Criminology International Journal*, *1*(3), 18.

7 Bird, S. R., Goebel, C., Burke, L. M. & Greaves, R. F. (2016). Doping in sport and exercise: anabolic, ergogenic, health and clinical issues. *Annals of Clinical Biochemistry*, *53*(2), 196–221.

8 Checker, D. I., Tracker, C. M. E. & Rabinovich, N. (2006). Anabolic androgenic steroids: A survey of 500 users. *Medicine and Science in Sports and Exercise*, *38*(4), 644–651.

9 Ip, E. J., Barnett, M. J., Tenerowicz, M. J. & Perry, P. J. (2012). Weightlifting's risky new trend: A case series of 41 insulin users. *Current Sports Medicine Reports*, *11*(4), 176–179.

10 Momaya, A., Fawal, M. & Estes, R. (2015). Performance-enhancing substances in sports: A review of the literature. *Sports Medicine*, *45*(4), 517–531.

11 Sagoe, D., Molde, H., Andreassen, C. S., Torsheim, T. & Pallesen, S. (2014). The global epidemiology of anabolic-androgenic steroid use: A meta-analysis and meta-regression analysis. *Annals of Epidemiology*, *24*(5), 383–398.

12 Grönbladh, A., Nylander, E. & Hallberg, M. (2016). The neurobiology and addiction potential of anabolic androgenic steroids and the effects of growth hormone. *Brain Research Bulletin*, *126*, 127–137.

13 Barghi, T. S., Halabchi, F., Dvorak, J. & Hosseinnejad, H. (2015). How the Iranian football coaches and players know about doping? *Asian Journal of Sports Medicine*, *6*(2), e24392–e24399.

14 Shuster. S. (2016). This is what Russia's doping scandal means for the Olympics, *Time | World*, 25 July. Sourced from http://time.com/4421019/russia-olympic-doping-report/

15 Brissonneau, C. (2006). Deviant careers: The case of cycling, In *Ethics and social science research in anti-doping*. WADA Conference, Larnaca, Cyprus, 13–14; Brissonneau C. (2010). Doping in France—1960–2000: American and Eastern Block influences. *Journal of Physical Education and Sport*, *27*(2), 33–39.

16 Assael, S. (2007). *Steroid Nation*. New York: ESPN.

17 Lentillon-Kaestner, L. & Carstairs, C. (2010). Doping among young elite cyclists: A qualitative psychosocial approach. *Scandinavian Journal of Medicine and Science in Sport*, *20*, 336–345.

18 Hunt, T. (2011). *Drug Games: The International Olympic Committee and the Politics of Doping*. Austin, TX: University of Texas Press; Hunt, T. (2007) Sports, drugs and the Cold War: The conundrum of Olympic doping policy 1970-1979. *Olympika: The International Journal of Olympic Studies International Centre for Olympic Studies*, 19–41.

19 Hunt, T. (2011). *Drug Games: The International Olympic Committee and the Politics of Doping*. Austin, TX: University of Texas Press, p.155.

20 Carlyon, P. (2005). Drugs in football. *The Bulletin*, 18 May, 12–16.

21 Robinson, M. (2002). Pot shots Lewis targeted after blowing whistle. *Herald Sun*, 7 March, 42.

22 Horvath, P. (2006). Anti-doping and human rights in sport: The case of the AFL and the WADA code. *Monash University Law Review*, *32*(2), 358–359.

23 Procon, D. (2011). Doping cases at the Olympics. Sourced from www.sportsanddrugs.procon.org/view.resource.php?resourceID=004420

24 Bahr, R. & Tjørnhom, M. (1998). Prevalence of doping in sports: doping control in Norway, 1977–1995. *Clinical Journal of Sport Medicine*, *8*(1), 32–37.

25 Mottram, D. (2011). The extent of doping in sport. In D. Mottram (ed.), *Drugs in sport (5th edn)*. London: Routledge, pp. 373–385; UK Sport (2005). Drug-free sport survey. London: UK Sport.

26 Pitsch, W. & Emrich, E. (2012). The frequency of doping in elite sport: Results of a replication study. *International Review for the Sociology of Sport*, *47*(5), 559–580; Striegel, H., Ulrich, R. & Simon, P. (2010). Randomized response estimates for doping and illicit drug use in elite athletes. *Drug and Alcohol Dependence*, *106*(2), 230–232.

27 Johnson, M. D., Jay, M. S., Shoup, B. & Rickert, V. I. (1989). Anabolic steroid use by male adolescents. *Pediatrics*, *83*(6), 921–924.

28 Tanner, S. M., Miller, D. W. & Alongi, C. (1995). Anabolic steroid use by adolescents: prevalence, motives, and knowledge of risks. *Clinical Journal of Sport Medicine*, *5*(2), 108–115.

29 Melia, P., Pipe, A. & Greenberg, L. (1996). The use of anabolic-androgenic steroids by Canadian students. *Clinical Journal of Sport Medicine*, *6*, 9–14.

30 Parkinson, A. B. & Evans, N. A. (2006). Anabolic androgenic steroids: A survey of 500 users. *Medicine & Science in Sports & Exercise*, *38*(4), 644–651.

31 Matilla, V., Rimplea, A., Jormanainen, V., Sahi, T. & Pihlajamaki, H. (2010) Anabolic-androgenic steroid use among young Finnish males. *Scandinavian Journal of Medicine and Science in Sports*, *20*, 330–335.

32 Wazaify, M., Bdair, A., Al-Hadidi, K. & Scott, J. (2014). Doping in gymnasiums in Amman: The other side of prescription and nonprescription drug abuse. *Substance Use & Misuse*, *49*(10), 1296–1302.

33 Striegal, H., Simon, P., Frisch, S., Roecker, K., Dietz, K., Dickhuth, H. & Ulrich, R. (2006). Anabolic ergogenic substance use in fitness-sport: A distinct group supported by the health care system. *Drug and Alcohol Dependence*, *81*, 11–19.

34 Anshel, M. (1991). A survey of elite athletes on the perceived causes of using banned drugs in sport. *Journal of Sport Behaviour*, *14*(4), 283–308.

35 Pearson, B. & Hansen, B. (1992). Survey of US Olympians. *USA Today*, 10C.

36 Laure, P. & Binsinger, C. (2005). Adolescent athletes and the demand and supply of drugs to improve performance. *Journal of Sports Science Medicine*, *4*, 272–277.

37 Cited in Cooper, C. (2012). *Run, Swim, Throw, Cheat: The Science Behind Drugs in Sport*. Oxford, UK: Oxford University Press.

38 Waddington, I. (2005). Changing patterns of drug use in British sport from the 1960s. *Sport in History*, *25*(3), 472–496.

39 Alaranta, A., Alaranta, H., Holmila, J., Palmu, P., Pietilä, K. & Helenius, I. (2006). Self-reported attitudes of elite athletes towards doping: Differences between types of sport. *International Journal of Sports Medicine*, *27*, 842–846.

40 Uvacsek, M., Nepusz, T., Naughton, D., Mazanov, J., Ranky, M. & Petroczi, A. (2009). Self-admitted behaviour and perceived use of performance–enhancing vs psychoactive drugs amongst competitive athletes. *Scandinavian Journal of Medicine and Science in Sport*, *16*, 111–131.

41 Dunn, M., Mazanov, J. & Sitharthan, A. (2009). Predicting future anabolic-androgenic steroid use intentions with current substance use: Findings from an internet-based survey. *Clinical Journal of Sports Medicine*, *19*(3), 222–227.

42 Moston, S., Skinner, J. & Engelberg, T. (2014). Perceived incidence of drug use in Australian sport: A survey of public opinion. *Sport in Society*, *15*(1), 64–72.

43 Kissalita, N. & Robinson, M. (2014). Attitudes and motivations of competitive cyclists regarding banned and legal performance enhancers. *Journal of Sport Science and Medicine*, *13*, 44–50.

44 Neeraj, K., Maman, P. & Sandhu, J. S. (2011). Why players engage in drug abuse substances. A survey study. *Doping Journal*, *8*, 1.

45 Court of Abritration for Sport (2015). CAS 2015/A/4059 World Anti-Doping Agency v. Thomas Bellchambers et al. Australian Football League, Australian Anti-Doping Authority.

46 Independent Commission (2015). Investigation Report #1 Final Report. Available at https://wada-main-prod.s3.amazonaws.com/resources/files/wada_independent_com mission_report_1_en.pdf (accessed 20 November 2015); Independent Commission. (2016). The Independent Commission Report #2. Available at https://wada-main-prod.s3.amazonaws.com/resources/files/wada_independent_commission_report_2_2016 _en.pdf (accessed 15 January 2016).

47 Peck, S., Vida, M. & Eccles, S. (2008). Adolescent pathways to adulthood drinking: sport activity involvement is not necessarily risky or protective. *Addiction*, *103* (1), 69–83.

48 Wichstrom, T. & Wichstrom, L. (2009) Does sport participation during adolescence prevent later alcohol, tobacco and cannabis use? *Addiction*, *104*, 138–149.

49 Spence, J. C. & Gauvin, L. (1996). Drug and alcohol use by Canadian university athletes: a national survey. *Journal of Drug Education*, *26*(3), 275–287.

50 Peretti-Watel, P., Guagloardp, V. Verger, P. & Pruvost, J. (2003). Sporting activity and drug use: Alcohol, cigarette and cannabis use among elite student athletes. *Addiction*, *98*, 1249–1256; Peretti-Watel, P., Beck, F. & Legleye, S. (2002). Beyond the u-curve: The relationship between sport and alcohol, cigarette and cannabis use in adolescents. *Addiction*, *97*(6), 707–716.

51 O'Malley, P. & Johnstone, I. (2001). Epidemiology of alcohol and other drug use among American college students. *Journal of Studies in Alcohol*, *14*, 23–39.

52 Wilson, G., Pritchard, M. & Shaffer, J. (2004). Athletic status and drinking behaviour in college students: The influence of gender and coping styles. *Journal of American College Health*, *52*(3), 269–273.

53 Ford, J. (2007). Substance use among college athletes: A comparison based on sport/team affiliation. *Journal of American College Health, 5*(6), 367–373.

54 Ford, J. (2007). Substance use among college athletes: A comparison based on sport/team affiliation. *Journal of American College Health, 5*(6), 367–373.

55 Ford, J. (2007) Substance use among college athletes: a comparison based on sport/team affiliation. *Journal of American College Health, 5*(6), 367–373.

56 Tahtamouni, L. H., Mustafa, N. H., Alfaouri, A. A., Hassan, I. M., Abdalla, M. Y. & Yasin, S. R. (2008). Prevalence and risk factors for anabolic-androgenic steroid abuse among Jordanian collegiate students and athletes. *The European Journal of Public Health, 18*(6), 661–665.

57 Dodge, T., Williams, K. J., Marzell, M. & Turrisi, R. (2012). Judging cheaters: is substance misuse viewed similarly in the athletic and academic domains? *Psychology of Addictive Behaviors, 26*(3), 678–682.

58 Karazsia, B. T., Crowther, J. H. & Galioto, R. (2013). Undergraduate men's use of performance-and appearance-enhancing substances: An examination of the gateway hypothesis. *Psychology of Men & Masculinity, 14*(2), 12–-137.

59 Duff, C., Scealy, M. & Rowland, B. (2004). The culture and context of alcohol use in community sporting clubs in Australia: Research into "attitudes" and "behavior". *Centre for Drug Studies, Australian Drug Foundation.*

60 Stilger, V. G. & Yesalis, C. E. (1999). Anabolic-androgenic steroid use among high school football players. *Journal of Community Health, 24*(2), 131–145.

61 Dunn, M. & White, V. (2011). The epidemiology of anabolic–androgenic steroid use among Australian secondary school students. *Journal of Science and Medicine in Sport, 14*(1), 10–14.

62 Rees, C., Zarco, E. & Lewis, D. (2009). The steroids/sports supplements connection: Pragmatism and sensation-seeking in the attitudes and behavior of JHS and HS students on Long Island. *Journal of Drug Education, 38*(4) 329–349.

63 Eisenberg, M. E., Wall, M. & Neumark-Sztainer, D. (2012). Muscle-enhancing behaviors among adolescent girls and boys. *Pediatrics, 136*(6), 1019–1026.

64 Goulet, C., Valois, P., Buist, A. & Côté, M. (2010). Predictors of the use of performance-enhancing substances by young athletes. *Clinical Journal of Sport Medicine, 20*(4), 243–248.

65 Thorlindsson, T. & Halldorsson, V. (2010). Sport, and use of anabolic androgenic steroids among Icelandic high school students: a critical test of three perspectives. *Substance Abuse: Treatment, Prevention, and Policy, 5*(1), 32.

66 Nolte, K., Steyn, B. J., Krüger, P. E. & Fletcher, L. (2016). Mindfulness, psychological well-being and doping in talented young high-school athletes. *South African Journal for Research in Sport, Physical Education and Recreation, 38*(2), 153–165.

67 Wanjek, B., Rosendahl, J., Strauss, B. & Gabriel, H. H. (2007). Doping, drugs and drug abuse among adolescents in the State of Thuringia (Germany): Prevalence, knowledge and attitudes. *International Journal of Sports Medicine, 28*(04), 346–353.

68 Veliz, P., Epstein-Ngo, Q., Austic, E., Boyd, C. & McCabe, S. E. (2015). Opioid use among interscholastic sports participants: an exploratory study from a sample of college students. *Research Quarterly for Exercise and Sport, 86*(2), 205–211.

69 Buckman, J. F., Farris, S. G. & Yusko, D. A. (2013). A national study of substance use behaviors among NCAA male athletes who use banned performance enhancing substances. *Drug and Alcohol Dependence, 131*(1), 50–55.

70 King, S., Carey, R. S., Jinnah, N., Millington, R., Phillipson, A., Prouse, C. & Ventresca, M. (2014). When is a drug not a drug? Troubling silences and unsettling painkillers in the National Football League. *Sociology of Sport Journal, 31*(3), 249–266.

71 King, S. (2014). Beyond the war on drugs? Notes on prescription opioids and the NFL. *Journal of Sport and Social Issues, 38*(2), 184–193.

72 Gruber, A. J. & Pope, H. G. (1998). Ephedrine abuse among 36 female weightlifters. *The American Journal on Addictions, 7*(4), 256–261.

73 Pope, H. G., Khalsa, J. H. & Bhasin, S. (2017). Body image disorders and abuse of anabolic-androgenic steroids among men. *JAMA, 317*(1), 23–24.

74 Mhillaj, E., Morgese, M. G., Tucci, P., Bove, M., Schiavone, S. & Trabace, L. (2015). Effects of anabolic-androgens on brain reward function. *Frontiers in Neuroscience*, *9*, 1–13.

75 Morente-Sánchez, J. & Zabala, M. (2013). Doping in sport: a review of elite athletes' attitudes, beliefs, and knowledge. *Sports Medicine*, *43*(6), 395–411.

76 Anshel, M. H. (1991). A survey of elite athletes on the perceived causes of using banned drugs in sport. *Journal of Sport Behavior*, *14*(4), 283.

77 Petrocelli, M., Oberweis, T. & Petrocelli, J. (2008). Getting huge, getting ripped: A qualitative exploration of recreational steroid use. *Journal of Drug Issues*, *38*(4), 1187–1205.

4

CHANNELS, CHOICES, CAUSES AND CODES

The impact of culture, values and ethnicity

Introduction

Drug use undeniably constitutes a problematic feature of sport and recreational activity around the world.[1] Of course, boosting performance with drugs can hardly be considered a new issue given that a variety of stimulants have been used to increase endurance since the late 19th century. However, the range of drugs now available, and their capacity to produce demonstrable and significant improvements, reflect a new suite of problems.[2] The various types and choices of muscle-building compounds, stimulants, blood-boosters and beta-blockers now available would fill an entire pharmacy. However, anabolic steroids, amphetamines and EPO reflect just the tip of the 'serious' PIEDS iceberg. We have noted the evidence suggesting that an array of licit and illicit drugs also receive liberal use for sporting and image purposes, ranging from alcohol, nicotine and narcotic analgesics to cocaine, cannabis, barbiturates and hallucinogenic cocktails.[3] In fact, as we mentioned earlier, alarmed sport officials concerned about the apparent increase in drug use imposed a raft of sanctions and prohibitions culminating in the establishment of WADA in 1999, and the publication of its inaugural Anti-Doping Code in 2004.

Numerous policy challenges, ideological issues and unanswered questions accompany the observations we just highlighted. The first question concerns to what extent PIEDS—and especially drug—use in sport occurs with more or less prevalence than in the broader community. The second question is to what extent this drug use varies between different sports. The third question is whether or not there are any significant variations within different sports.

To the first question, many commentators intuitively answer that drug use in sport will occur less frequently than in general society due to its emphasis on getting the most out of the body, and fine-tuning it to achieve optimum performance. Moreover, a strong groundswell of opinion proclaims that sport provides a sanctuary against drug use because of the values it inculcates into its participants. It does this by: 1) demanding conformity; 2) ensuring close supervision; 3) producing bonding and cohesion; and 4) providing a structured forum for displays of masculinity. According to Eitle et al., sport lessens the need for young men, in particular, to create an identity on the back of anti-social and deviant behaviours. As a result, it builds character and a more reflective personality, which in turn, lead to lower levels of alcohol and drug use.[4]

Off-the-cuff answers to the second question acknowledge that different sports and games require unique structures and organisation, and revere distinctive histories and traditions. These differences produce practices and cultures where different skills, physical capabilities and personalities are required to ensure high levels of performance. For example, highly combative sports like football and boxing demand severe levels of aggression, while more aesthetic and technical sports like gymnastics and equestrianism encourage precision and control. Taking a further step in the argument, aggressive and combative sports necessitate higher levels of drug use. Furthermore, sport's commercial scale affects drug use levels where performance pressure escalates in sports where player salaries are high, and extensive wagering takes place on the outcome of the game or event. It would also be reasonable to expect quite different cultures to be built around high-risk sports like ultimate fighting and motorcycle racing, on the one hand, and low-risk sports like lawn bowls and darts on the other.

A reflexive response to the third question predicts significant differences among sports. Players and athletes do not grow up in a social and cultural vacuum, but rather import attitudinal and behavioural baggage that has been accumulated through their personality development, family upbringing, adherence to ethnic expectations, the re-telling and ceremonial re-enactment of cultural traditions, schooling experiences, the influence of peers and the impact of religious education and socialisation. Additional influences arise as gender expectations and class distinctions play out. It would therefore be expected, for example, that athletes raised in strict households underpinned by strong religious and/or moral convictions would be less likely to use drugs than athletes bought up in libertarian households where parents exercised ambivalence about strict moral codes and organised religion.[5]

Another interesting question considers how competing values play out in practice. Will, for instance, the values embedded in a player's ethnic identity override the customs and beliefs built into a particular sport club or sporting community? Or alternatively, does a player's core personality or sense of gender identity establish the main behavioural cues when decisions need to be made about using or not using certain drugs in a sport setting? Despite the salience of these questions, little research examines the ways in which ethnicity, cultural traditions and religion influence drug use in sport or in the broader recreational community. However, solid evidence indicates that in the wider community, ethno-cultural factors mediate drug use in a number of important ways. For example, in a 2001 study of American high school students undertaken by

Marsiglia et al., respondents who self-identified as African- and Mexican-American had the lowest reported levels of drug use, while those respondents who self-identified as white had the highest usage levels.[6] Miller-Day and Barnett replicated these results in 2004, reporting that nearly 51% of white respondents aged 12 years and over had used alcohol in the past 12 months compared with 34% of African-Americans. The 2003 study by Eitle et al. on college students also revealed higher levels of alcohol consumption by white respondents than by African-American respondents.[7]

A 2007 survey of illicit drug use by McCabe et al. highlighted differences between various ethnic groups in a sample of US college students.[8] Where the level of usage for cannabis amongst women was highest for white respondents and Hispanics, it fell to 25% for African-Americans and 23% for Asians. While the illicit (non-prescription) use of pain medication drugs was lower for all female groups, significant differences appeared between ethnic groups. The highest level was recorded by Hispanic respondents, who reported a 10% usage level, while the lowest was amongst Asian respondents, who claimed a 3% usage level. Illicit stimulant medication usage ranged from just over 7% for white and Hispanic respondents to a low of 1% for African-Americans. Similar inter-ethnic differences appeared for college men, although the overall levels of use exceeded female rates. For example, while the usage level of cannabis was 46% for Hispanics and 43% for white respondents, it fell to 34% for African-Americans and 28% for Asians. For pain medication the highest usage level was 9% for white respondents, while the lowest was 5% for Asians and African-Americans. Finally, the usage level of stimulant medication varied from 9% for Hispanics to 4% for Asians.

An earlier study by Bachman et al. discovered the same kinds of differences based around ethnicity.[9] High school students who used alcohol at least once in the previous 12 months reached a high for white males and females at around 88%, with Mexican- and Native American males not far behind at just over 82%. The lowest percentage usage occurred in the African-American female and Native American female cohorts, at 64% and 61%, respectively. The variation in use was equally pronounced for cannabis. Whereas 42% of Native American males, 40% of white males and 38% of Mexican-American males had used cannabis in the last 12 months, the usage rates for Asian males, African-American males and Asian males was 20%, 18% and 17%, respectively.

Some gaps can be seen in the ethno-cultural evidence base. For example, the limited empirical data say little about sport-related correlations, and at this point it remains unclear what differences occur in sport settings. One of the few studies examining the interplay of sport affiliation and ethno-cultural identity was undertaken by Eitle et al.,[10] which noted a marginally greater level of drug use amongst young adult white males, as well as a significantly greater level of alcohol use. We can speculate on a number of possible explanations. First, perhaps playing high school sport for this cohort is a kind of gateway to a hyper-masculine subculture. Second, perhaps these results reinforce, as Bloom et al. noted as early as 1997, a tradition of young white men following football, accompanied by a strong drinking culture.[11] Finally, perhaps the data reflect higher levels of alcohol consumption amongst white males in the wider society.

When it comes to proclaiming relationships between drug use—especially PEDS and ethnicity, religiosity and cultural traditions—we should proceed carefully. The results of studies in this area are illuminating, but they do not directly tackle the question of exactly how ethno-cultural identity impacts upon drug use in a sporting context, and to what extent the values and culture of sport clubs or associations will supersede the values, customs and norms that different ethno-cultural groups bring with them to their sporting practices. Many research gaps remain to be filled. We need additional research to determine just how strongly sport club cultures support, and even encourage drug use activities, and whether sports participation actually increases drug and alcohol use.

Determinants of PIEDS use and intervention approaches

The problematic nature of the PIEDS issue raises questions about why some athletes and players willingly jeopardise their sporting careers and well-being by sidestepping anti-doping codes and/or ignoring health warnings, and use PIEDS without proper supervision and with only a smattering of knowledge. Despite all the talk around the moral and health dangers associated with uncontrolled drug use in sport,[12] and the hostile view that most observers hold about drug use in sport,[13] we still have only a meagre knowledge of the attitudes, values and motivations of sportspeople who employ various substances to boost performance, build their physique, relieve stress and lighten moods. In the context of non-elite or recreational sport, we know even less. Yet understanding athlete and sport participant attitudes and behaviours around PIEDS should be the foundation upon which to construct effective policy,[14] interventions and educational programmes.

An extensive review of the literature on doping attitudes, influences and interventions, focusing on both elite and non-elite athletes, reveals that despite a growth in research, significant gaps in knowledge remain. Based on this review, it was concluded that: 1) PIEDS use occurs within a complex system of socio-demographic and psychosocial predictors; 2) critical incidents within and outside of sport can increase vulnerability to dangerous PIEDS use; 3) reference groups, such as peers and coaches, can play a key role in encouraging or discouraging various forms of PIEDS practice; 4) the detection of illegal and banned PIEDS use is generally perceived to be low; and 5) exposure to PIEDS education is inadequate, as is the level of knowledge surrounding the effects of use.[15]

More generally, it is somewhat ironic that sport participation is not always an antidote to recreational drug and substance use. In fact, the opposite is often the case. Research has shown that young people who play competitive sport may engage in more drug and alcohol use than those who play little organised sport.[16] Some evidence even reveals that substance use correlates to engagement in other high-risk consumption behaviours.[17] For example, as we observed earlier, studies of college students in the United States found that those involved in athletics engaged in more risky behaviours than non-athletes,[18] with a particular preference for binge-drinking.[19] Moreover, the focus in sport on team-bonding on the one hand, and intensive competition on the other, makes it fertile ground for the growth of drug use and abuse.

The following discussion focuses on the use of PIEDS in sport, and where possible, highlights research in the context of non-elite sport, including information on the limited intervention and education programmes that currently exist. It provides an overview of what is currently known about the attitudes and perceptions, contextual influences and personal characteristics of individuals in relation to the use of PIEDS, and how governments and sporting associations have responded. Exposing the pressures and factors that influence attitudes and behaviours can help to inform educational approaches that may modify athletes' (recreational, developing or elite) propensities to take image and performance enhancing substances, or at least minimise the harm for those determined to do so. Such information is critical to the development of effective intervention and education programmes, especially given that they are in scant supply at the recreational and community levels.

Contextual influences on athlete attitudes and use of PIEDS

Athletes are often reticent to reveal their views on substance use in sport.[20] As a result, it is unclear how attitudes to PIEDS are initially formulated, what factors have influenced those attitudes over athletes' formative years, and the contextual and cultural factors that may have shaped their attitudes during their playing careers. A much-cited study[21] identified six inputs that influence changes in the attitude-behaviour of athletes towards PEDS. These were: 1) threat appraisal, reflecting the deterrence factor or the cost of being caught; 2) incentive appraisal, representing the benefits of drug use; 3) reference group opinions, highlighting the importance of peer approval; 4) personal morality, illustrating an athlete's views on right and wrong; 5) the perceived legitimacy of the drug authority's position; and, 6) personality factors, which are individualised variables linked to self-esteem and optimism.

Consistent with the theory of planned behaviour,[22] this study made two central assumptions. First, behaviour is basically rational and that athletes use information in a systematic manner to inform their decisions about drug use. Second, athletes consider the implications of their behaviour before they act. These twin assumptions represent a kind of rational intentionality, but they may not always be satisfied in practice, and consequently predictions about behaviour based on these factors alone will most probably be compromised.

In contrast, the importance of coercion, punishments and the risk of getting caught were the focus of another study[23] that analysed behaviours involving PEDS. Using the concept of deterrence, which has its theoretical basis in criminal decision making, this research specified four categories of salience. The first was legal sanctions, which can take the form of fines and suspensions. The second was social sanctions, which includes disapproval, ostracism by friends and colleagues, and potential material losses from sponsors who may elect to find someone else to endorse their products. The third was self-imposed sanctions that are bound up in the guilt, loss of face and plummeting self-worth arising from being publicly identified as a cheat. The final category was health concern from the likely side effects associated with the chronic use of a specific drug. These costs and sanctions are then weighed against the benefits that might arise from the use of PEDS.

Players and athletes are subject to the values, belief and practices of their sporting colleagues.[24] Their attitudes about substance use consequently form within a defined context where situational factors and the behaviour of coaches, peers, friends and team-mates represent powerful influences on their attitudes and practices. Furthermore, data suggest that attitudes are contingent upon the ease of access to the substance, its performance impact and the substance's social acceptance.[25]

In general, the use of banned performance enhancing substances is viewed as cheating, although for different reasons between elite and non-elite athletes, with non-elite players and athletes being more moralistic. The use of 'hard' non-performance enhancing recreational or illicit substances is viewed as foolish, but not morally reprehensible, by non-elite and elite players and athletes alike, while the use of legal non-performance enhancing substances is acceptable to just about everyone. While many non-elite athletes may eschew illegal substances, their knowledge of these agents is limited as is their understanding of legal over-the-counter medications and nutritional supplements. Regarding the latter, the legality and availability of these substances through reputable sources can eliminate the perception of risk.[26]

When reflecting on our own studies of players and athletes, and studies of drug use in sport undertaken by other researchers, it appears that attitudes and use are shaped by far more than an individual calculation of the weighted costs and benefits of using and not being caught, using and being caught, not using and being caught, and not using and not being caught. The influences on player and athlete practices are both multifactorial and subjectively interpreted. They begin with the impact of micro factors that include a mix of intra- and interpersonal influences that shape personal identities and their subsequent expression. They move onto a range of so-called external forces that include people with expertise, authority and a charismatic presence on one hand, and the rewards and benefits that come from achieving excellence on the other. Each receives attention in the following sections.

Personality and identity

While at a societal level an individual's personality and sense of identity influences behaviour,[27] the research evidence fails to conclusively highlight any specific traits and dispositions that correspond to attitudes about drug use in sport. Contemporary studies do not reveal any clear-cut association between a self-identified temperament, gender identity, life experience or moral code and a particular position on substance use in sport. Although these factors appear to be intuitively relevant, particularly gender, it remains unclear as to how they affect attitude formation around drug use in sport. One recurring theme, however, is the self-driven nature of elite athletes and their early awareness of a single-minded desire to excel that had been evident from childhood. Recent studies[28] have also shown that young people with high emotional intelligence ratings—which means they have a strong capacity for self-awareness, empathy and impulse control—are likely to be low users of cannabis and alcohol, although results are not explicitly related to sport.

In the context of adolescent sport, there is evidence to suggest that males are more prone to PEDS use, as are those athletes with lower self-esteem or with a lower ability to resist social pressure.[29] Conversely, the following protective factors against doping have been identified in the context of college or university athletes: a strong moral stance; self-control; having an identity beyond sport; resilience to social group pressure; and, secure attachments outside of sport.[30]

People of influence

Five categories of influential people shape the ways in which athletes—particularly the young—make their way through the sporting world, and may directly or indirectly provide the impetus for substance use. They are: 1) family; 2) peers; 3) teachers; 4) coaches; and 5) heroes. Adult mentors influence players and athletes during their sporting careers, and their attitudes to substance use are partly shaped by these relationships. Parents, and particularly fathers, loom large, playing instrumental roles in shaping their children's sport-career paths, a view consistent with previous work in sport development studies.[31] However, parental influences are not necessarily positive. Fathers can be excessively ambitious for their children, pressuring them to become highly competitive. For elite athletes, the most important influencers are coaches, usually the first elite-level coach.[32] Coaches are seen as not only inspirational and knowledgeable, but also to be obeyed without question.

Early sporting experiences

In concert with influential people, critical early sporting experiences also shape attitudes towards substances, with the key issues including the places where athletes grew up, the sports they participated in and the level of competition they played in.[33] The more frequently the early experiences of players and athletes emphasised serious competition, the more likely those players and athletes would hold permissive attitudes towards both licit and illicit performance enhancing substances.

Commercial pressures

Amongst the commercial pressures impacting upon attitudes to substance use, the most prominent are professionalisation, sponsorship, rewards and fame. These factors help explain the pressure to use performance enhancing substances for elite athletes, or for those aspiring to that status. Financial incentives tempt players and athletes to use various substances, whether available over the counter, secured by prescription or obtained through illegal trafficking. Some empirical studies[34] on the impact of commercial incentives on player and athlete behaviour have highlighted similar issues. The drive to secure a competitive edge is strongest where the rewards—psychic, social or financial—are the highest.

Sporting culture

No one single sporting culture exists, even within a single sport or competition. A sport's culture—its prevailing values and beliefs—is built around several common features, which nearly always include masculinity, risk taking and aggressiveness. The prominence of these features will, in turn, influence a participant's attitudes towards substance use. Values and beliefs form in complex ways, unique to individual sports and influenced by not only the above factors, but also by the physical performance requirements of the sport. A sport's demands can focus on power and strength (e.g. weightlifting), endurance and stamina (e.g. triathlon) or technical skill (e.g. sailing). It can sometimes also involve a distinctive combination of all three (e.g. gymnastics). Other features that can shape a sport's culture include the level at which it is performed (i.e. elite or non-elite), whether the sport is team or individually based, its level of medicalisation and scientisation, and the degree to which it values social engagement over success and winning.

Given the different ways in which sport activities can be structured and organised, the radical cultural differences hardly seem surprising. For example, elite cycling involves strong medical and scientific support, including a heavy reliance on physicians, support therapists, sport scientists, biomechanists and engineers.[35] For professional cyclists, licit performance enhancing substances like caffeine, analgesics and nutritional supplements present a way of life—essential for completing long and gruelling road races, and an accepted part of the culture of professional competition. Another example can be found in football codes where, at the non-elite level in particular, the social club, being the distribution point for alcoholic beverages, is a focal point for building camaraderie and ensuring social cohesion. This emphasis on networking and investing in social capital is accompanied by a heavy drinking culture that includes a few weekly beers at one end of the continuum, and regular binge-drinking at the other.

Attitudes to substance use in sport

Most serious athletes concede that drug use of one sort or another constitutes an ongoing feature of their chosen sports.[36] Substances have been used in sport over a long period of time, although in recent years the varieties of substances, and their potency in improving performance, have increased significantly. In relation to PIEDS, our own research indicates that non-elite athletes are far more rigid and moralistic in their views than their professional and high performing counterparts.[37] Non-elite athletes tend to agree with the WADA's policy platform on performance enhancing substances, maintaining that athletes should not be allowed to utilise drugs that artificially bolster performances, harm their health or undermine the 'spirit of sport'. While non-elite athletes seem comfortable with stronger penalties for transgressors, we found that elite athletes take a more practical approach towards performance enhancing substances, where banned equates to 'wrong' and legal represents an 'opportunity'. For example, strong painkillers and some narcotic analgesics are acceptable, along with caffeine, because they are not banned, even though dosages might be unhealthy and potentially dangerous.

For elite athletes, moral issues are not particularly relevant, which partly explains why their attitudes appear to be disconnected from their personality or identity. Elite athletes see themselves operating in a sporting culture supporting the use of medical treatments and substances to sustain performance. Furthermore, coaches and managers have a vested interest in getting injured athletes back on to the field of play in the shortest possible time, and may employ a cocktail of painkilling and anti-inflammatory drugs to speed up the process. Earlier studies have similarly found that athletes receive their first substances from trusted sources close to them.[38]

Any analysis of attitudes to substances in sport begs the questions as to how these attitudes were formed in the first place, and what were the major factors that shaped them. As noted earlier, player and athlete attitude formation about drugs in sport is a complex amalgam of factors, incorporating sporting culture, its commercial scale, the influence of others, critical incidents experienced through the player and athlete life-cycle and the level at which players perform their sport.

Critical incidents and experiences, in particular, play a crucial role in forming and strengthening attitudes, which in part explains the ways in which athletes' attitudes differ between different PIEDS types. For elite athletes a return from injury, selection to a representative team, overcoming a previous failure or meeting a sponsor goal may be crucial in continuing in their chosen professions. While non-elite athletes do not necessarily face such make-or-break scenarios, peer pressure, a desire to be seen as a 'winner' and the increasingly competitive nature of so-called recreational sport all produce their own moments where goals and commitment to achievement come to the forefront, and actions as pronounced as seeking help from drugs can materialise.

Such observations offer lessons for strategic interventions at pivotal moments in athletes' decision-making life cycles. In this context, we suggest a re-visit to a model suggested by Petroczi and Aidman in a study published in 2008.[39] It suggests that deterrence strategies focusing on the use of prohibited substances are less effective than those initiatives targeting contextual factors at the career stages of athletes' professional lives when they are most vulnerable to external influences.

This model highlights the influence of situational factors, facilitating an environment where doping-related decisions are influenced by a complex intersection of trait, systemic and situational factors related to goal setting and achievement.

This model also predicts that many of those factors that either motivate or enable use can also operate as constraints. For example, a personality that shuns risky behaviour, a moralistic club culture and the imposition of sanctions for deviance may inhibit substance use.[40]

PIEDS interventions in community and non-elite sport

Reports exploring the use of PIEDS in various countries have indicated that the use of these substances in the context of community or recreational sport is of growing concern. The use and abuse of PIEDS is also widely acknowledged as an area that has been overshadowed by the focus on elite and professional sport. A report on doping prevention by the European Commission in 2014 cited that two-thirds of its member states characterised the prevention of doping in recreational sport as important or very important, and more broadly, that the 'misuse of doping agents in recreational sport has become a societal problem and a public health issue that must be addressed'.[41]

Within Australia—a leader in the area and a salient case study—calls for better education and intervention in matters regarding 'sport drugs' have been made by medical authorities and leaders within the sport community, citing the perceived and documented rise of supplement use (both legal and illegal) as of immense concern.[42] Much of the policy work, including education and intervention, has been undertaken by the Australian Sports Anti-Doping Authority (ASADA[43]) and the Department of Health's National Integrity of Sport Unit (NISU[44]), and is embedded within broader government policies on healthy behaviours. This issue has also been acknowledged at the state government level. For example, the Victorian State Government has an 'Anti-Doping Policy' that speaks to the need for a culture free of drugs while also emphasising the role of non-elite sport in reflecting fairly obtained athletic achievement.[45] A major initiative aimed at tackling illicit drug use in sport and in the community was undertaken in 2009, when the Australian Federal Government contributed funding (over $20 million) to prepare the 'Illicit Drugs in Sport—National Education and Prevention Action Plan'.

While ASADA and NISU remain the pre-eminent anti-doping bodies in Australia, other groups play a key role. For example, Sports Medicine Australia (SMA), an umbrella organisation for sport science and medicine, have had branches in Victoria (via CleanEdge) and Western Australia (via BeDrugFree) providing training and resources in community-based PIEDS education. However, in recent years, these programmes appear to have fallen by the wayside, relegating the responsibility to ASADA and the NISU.

There has been some attempt to introduce new approaches that sit alongside these organisations to help broach education and intervention at community levels, targeting children specifically. A 2013 report,[46] by sport consultancy Bluestone Edge, suggested that a diversified approach could implement and deliver a national education programme in Australia to bridge a gap between ASADA, the NISU, the community and various support agencies (including sporting organisations). However, the proposal has not yet fully eventuated. One support agency is 'Play by the Rules',[47] a group founded in 2001 with the broad mandate to focus on the sporting behaviours of children. Play by the Rules released three videos[48] and an e-book,[49] via their website, covering the topic of supplements at the community sport level, perhaps reflecting the increased awareness of this issue. The initiative also corresponds to a recommendation from the Bluestone Edge report that Play by the Rules should be 'promoted throughout the network as an advocacy-based central program that delivers resources, multi-media education, CSA/social media campaigns and forums on anti-doping, illicit drugs and supplements to sub-elite and grassroots sport'.[50]

The ASADA intervention programmes are aimed primarily at aspiring athletes, and offer two levels of anti-doping education through an e-learning portal.[51] In addition, lesson plans and materials are available for use in secondary schools[52] (Years 9–12) covering five topic areas, four of which relate directly to PIEDS: Integrity and Anti-Doping in Sport, Anti-Doping in Sport, Illicit Drugs in Sport and Ethics and Ethical Decision Making in Sport. These materials are complemented by information offered by the NISU through their 'Illicit Drugs in Sport Program', which aims to provide guidance to athletes, coaches and administrators when faced with illicit drug issues in their sports. Online courses exist for athletes, coaches, sport officers and presenters.[53]

More broadly, the landscape of international programmes aimed at PIEDS intervention lacks a central repository to facilitate best practice, and lacks any rigorous assessment of sustainable impact. A detailed study by the Institute for Sport, Physical Activity and Leisure at Leeds Beckett University,[54] prepared for WADA, makes for informative, yet alarming, reading. It highlights the limited number of studies that consider the effectiveness of intervention programmes.[55] In addition, the studies were concentrated within a narrow geographic and demographic segment. Of the 17 studies presenting programme results since the 1990s, nine focused on high school settings within the US. The result is not surprising given that the longest-running programs are US based: 'Athletes Training & Learning to Avoid Steroids' (ATLAS) and 'Athletes Targeting Healthy Exercise & Nutrition Alternatives' (ATHENA). (Both ATLAS and ATHENA were developed by the Oregon Health & Science University.)

ATLAS is targeted toward males, while ATHENA focuses on females. Both offer peer-led training through 8–10 sessions of 45 minutes. While these two programmes remain the most researched interventions,[56] a meta-analysis of the limited studies in this field suggest they, like other programmes, presently offer only marginal reductions in doping intentions, but no significant change to doping behaviour; correlates of doping intentions and behaviours were unsurprisingly: 1) using legal supplements; 2) perceived social norms; and 3) favourable attitudes towards doping.[57]

In the UK, online guidance, similar to the training programmes offered by ASADA/NISU, is provided by the UK Anti-Doping (UKAD) organisation, a 'Non-Departmental Public Body' accountable to the British parliament via the Department for Culture, Media and Sport. Its education programmes[58] are specifically designed for the 'beginner to elite' level and include pathways for parents, coaches, support personnel and education partners. The '100% ME' programme in this domain is one of the few such regimes outside of the US to have been evaluated, although in this instance the study was tangential to the outcomes of the programme as it focused on the role of tutors who administer anti-doping information.[59]

Intervention studies

The Leeds Beckett report[60] identified that, between 2007 and 2015, only eight studies had investigated the effects of anti-doping education or intervention programmes. These were spread geographically across the US (three studies), the UK (two studies), with others in France, Germany and Iran.

The US studies focused on the ATHENA programme noted previously and on an intervention programme termed SATURN (Student Athlete Testing Using Random Notification) with results indicating a minimal impact. One ATHENA study[61] on over 1600 female athletes who participated in eight sessions of 45 minutes each that were integrated into team meetings by coaches, identified some initial impact on potential steroid use, but this had dissipated within nine months. A similar study on athletes (n=368) across nine schools using a longer follow-up period (one to three years after high school graduation) indicated reduced marijuana and alcohol use, although there was no difference between the intervention and control group in the use of other substances, including ecstasy, LSD and diet pills and diuretics.[62] The SATURN study,[63] which compared students in schools containing a random drug and alcohol testing policy, with a control group of schools, found that the potential deterrence of a structured testing programme had minimal effect, with no differences between groups at multiple follow-up points for illicit drug or alcohol usage. Of concern, however, was the suggestion that students at the schools with the policy initiatives had higher negative attitudes toward the purpose and benefits of testing.

The two UK studies were relatively specific. One study[64] evaluated the '100% me' program, which aims to provide anti-doping information and education through a network of tutors in the UK. As the study looked at the role of the tutors and not the impact of their work, it is hard to form any clear judgement as to its efficacy, despite the positive intentions of the programme. The other UK-based study[65] targeted male gym patrons using a leaflet intervention. It indicated some effect on food knowledge through this process. The study also reinforced the notion that the Internet and training partners are the key sources of information with regard to enhancement products.

Potentially showing some impact of interventions were more recent studies conducted in Germany, France and Iran. The latter study[66] also considered male, recreational gym users, noting that approximately half of the respondents indicated that their coaches and/or friends were steroid users, with the goal of enhancing attractiveness far outweighing that of improving athletic performance. An intervention programme, using a variety of methods including audio-visual CDs, group discussion and leaflets, had an impact on intention to use steroids; however, after intervention, actual use did not decline. The study[67] in Germany focused on young elite athletes, using a relatively novel quasi-experimental design whereby participants worked through a series of ethical doping dilemmas and provided written responses. The results of this study indicated that the decision-making approach used was successful in breaking up stereotypical reasoning about doping, although the value of this on usage is not yet fully established. The final study,[68] based in France, showed a moderate impact on young students (aged 10–11) and those who participated in sport more than 10 hours per week, following information sessions on self-medication and activities related to building self-assertion.

The narrow evidence noted here is further hampered by limitations in methods and design implementation. There appears to be a considerable reliance on self-reporting and difficulty in identifying user bases for testing, particularly among recreational participants. There also appears to be a priority on measuring change in attitude and/or intentions, rather than on athlete behaviour. Overall, the studies provide limited evidence of cause and effect, which restricts their use in establishing government policy and protection protocols. It is easy to concur here with the Leeds Beckett study that there is a significant 'absence of evidence' about the efficacy of intervention programmes.[69]

Conclusion

The evidence has mounted concerning the considerable health risks associated with PIEDS, particularly by adolescents who are engaged in social or competitive sport and who seek to 'better' their performance (or reflect their idols) in order to attain some form of gratification or reward.[70] Complicating factors include the assumption that medical-style intervention programmes (where considerable research exists—for example in tobacco consumption) are not necessarily easily applicable, given the intricate human behaviours associated with sporting and recreational participation that extend beyond the dysfunctional or pathological. PIEDS usage, with regard to legal substances, may already be normalised within certain groups where peer pressure or consumptive practices to enable winning are the prime consideration. Nevertheless, a 'systems-based' approach may be applicable that emphasises education and can cut across the myriad of complicating factors relevant to non-elite users of PIEDS. This would need to draw on high levels of collaboration, a commitment to inter-disciplinary work across multiple sites and contexts and concerted efforts to combine theory with practice to ensure a translation of methods that can readily be implemented.[71]

Notes

1 Pound, R. W. (2008). *Inside Dope: How Drugs are the Biggest Threat to Sports, Why you Should Care, and What can be Done about Them*. Ontario, CA: John Wiley; Simon, P., Striegel, H., Aust, F., Dietz, K. & Ulrich, R. (2006). Doping in fitness sports: estimated number of unreported cases and individual probability of doping. *Addiction, 101*(11), 1640–1644.

2 Backhouse, S., McKenna, J. & Patterson, L. (2007). Prevention through education: A review of current international social science literature—A focus on the prevention of bullying, tobacco, alcohol, and social drugs use in children, adolescents and young adults. World Anti-Doping Agency/Carnegie Research Institute, Leeds University; Backhouse, S., McKenna, J., Robinson, S., & Atkin, A. (2007). *Attitudes, Behaviours, Knowledge and Education—Drugs in Sport: Past, Present and Future*. Montreal, QC: World Anti-Doping Agency; Cooper, C. (2012). *Run, Swim, Throw, Cheat: The Science Behind Drugs in Sport*. Oxford, UK: Oxford University Press; Hanstad, D. (2009). Sport, health, and drugs: A critical re-examination of some key issues and problems. *Perspectives in Public Health, 129*(4), 174–182.

3 Pampel, F. (2007). *Drugs and Sport*. New York: Infobase; Parisotto, R. (2006). *Blood Sports: The Inside Dope on Drugs in Sport*. Melbourne: Hardie Grant.

4 Eitle, D., McNulty, J. & Eitle, T. (2003). The deterrence hypothesis re-examined: Sports participation and substance abuse among young adults. *Journal of Drug Issues, 33*(1), 193–222.

5 Richard, A. J., Bell, D. C. & Carlson, J. W. (2000). Individual religiosity, moral community, and drug user treatment. *Journal for the Scientific Study of Religion, 39*(2), 240–246.

6 Marsiglia, F., Kulis, S. & Hecht, M. (2001). Ethnic labels and ethnic identity as predictors of drug use amongst middle school students in the southwest. *Journal of Research on Adolescents, 11*(1), 21–48.

7 Eitle, D., McNulty, J. & Eitle, T. (2003). The deterrence hypothesis re-examined: Sports participation and substance abuse among young adults. *Journal of Drug Issues, 33*(1), 193–222.

8 McCabe, S., Morales, M. Cranford, J., Delva, J., McPherson, M. & Boyd, C. (2007). Race/ethnicity and gender differences in drug use and abuse among college students. *Journal of Ethnicity in Substance Abuse, 6*(2), 75–95.

9 Bachman, J., Wallace, J., O'Malley, P., Johnstone, L., Kurth, C & Neighbors, K. (1991). Racial/ethnic differences in smoking, drinking and illicit drug use among American high school seniors. *American Journal of Public Health, 81*(3), 372–377.

10 Eitle, D., McNulty, J. & Eitle, T. (2003). The deterrence hypothesis re-examined: Sports participation and substance abuse among young adults. *Journal of Drug Issues, 33*(1), 193–222.

11 Bloom, P., Hogan, J. & Blazing, J. (1997). Sports promotion and teen smoking and drinking. *American Journal of Health Behaviour, 21*, 100–109.

12 Ingram, S. (2004). Buff enough? *Current Science, 90*(2), 4–5; Parisotto, R. (2006). *Blood Sports: The Inside Dope on Drugs in Sport*. Melbourne: Hardie Grant.

13 Moston, S., Skinner, J. & Engelberg, T. (2012) Perceived incidence of drug use in Australian sport: A survey of public opinion, *Sport in Society, 15*(1), 64–72.

14 British Medical Association (2002). Policy Instruments to prevent the use of drugs in sport, in *Drugs in Sport: The Pressure to Perform*. London: British Medical Association.

15 Leeds Beckett Institute for Sport, Physical Activity and Leisure (2015). *Social Psychology of Doping in Sport: A Mixed-studies Narrative Synthesis*. Montreal, QC: World Anti-Doping Agency.

16 Ford, J. (2007). Substance use among college athletes: A comparison based on sport/team affiliation, *Journal of American College Health, 5*(6), 367–373; Hildebrand, K., Johnson, D. & Bogle, K. (2001). Comparisons of patterns of alcohol use between high school and college athletes and non-athletes, *College Studies Journal, 45*(6), 358–365.

17 Laure, P. & Binsinger, C. (2005). Adolescent athletes and the demand and supply of drugs to improve performance, *Journal of Sports Science Medicine*, 4, 272–277; Wiefferink, C., Detmar, S., Coumans, B. Vogels, T. & Paulussen, T. (2008). Social psychological determinants of the use of performance-enhancing drugs by gym users, *Health Education Research*, 23(1), 70–80.

18 Selby, R., Weinstein, H. & Bird, T. (1990). The health of university athletes: attitudes, behaviors and stressors. *Journal of American College Health*, 39(1), 11–18.

19 Wechsler, H., Davenport, A., Dowdell, G., Grossman, S. & Zanakos, S. (1997). Binge drinking, tobacco and illegal drug use and involvement in athletics: a survey of students at 140 American colleges. *Journal of American College Health*, 21(4), 195–200.

20 Petróczi, A. (2007). Attitudes and doping: A structural equation analysis of the relationship between athletes' attitudes, sport orientation and doping behaviour. *Substance Abuse Treatment, Prevention, and Policy*, 2(34), 1–15; Petroczi, A. & Aidman, E. (2008). Psychological drivers in doping: The life-cycle model of performance enhancement. *Substance Abuse Treatment, Prevention, and Policy*, 3(7), 3–12.

21 Donovan, R. J., Egger, G., Kapernick, V. & Mendoza, J. (2002). A conceptual framework for achieving performance enhancing drug compliance in sport, *Sports Medicine*, 32(4), 269–284.

22 Ajzen, I. (1991). The theory of planned behaviour, *Organizational Behavior and Human Decision Processes, 50*, 179–211; Ajzen, I. & Fishbein, M. (1980). *Understanding Attitudes and Predicting Social Behaviour*. Englewood Cliffs, NJ: Prentice-Hall.

23 Strelan, P. & Boeckmann, R. (2003). A new model for understanding performance-enhancing drug use by elite athletes. *Journal of Applied Sport Psychology*, 15, 176–183.

24 Petroczi, A. & Aidman, E. (2008). Psychological drivers in doping; The life-cycle model of performance enhancement. *Substance Abuse Treatment, Prevention, and Policy*, 3(7), 3–12.

25 Smith, A., Stewart, B., Oliver-Bennetts, S., McDonald, S., Ingerson, L., Anderson, A., Dickson, G., Emery, P. & Graetz, F. (2010). Contextual influences and athlete attitudes to drugs in sport. *Sport Management Review*, 13(3), 181–197.

26 Henning, A. (2014). (Self-)surveillance, anti-doping and health in non-elite running. *Surveillance & Society*, 11, 494–507.

27 Burke, P. & Stets, J. (2009). *Identity Theory*, Oxford, UK: Oxford University Press; Burstyn, V. (1999). *The Rites of Men: Manhood, Politics, and the Culture of Sport*. Toronto, ON: University of Toronto Press; Mittal, B. (2006). I, me, and mine—how products become consumer's extended selves. *Journal of Consumer Behaviour*, 5, 550–562.

28 Claros, E. & Sharma, M. (2010). The relationship between emotional intelligence and abuse of alcohol, marijuana and tobacco among college students, *Journal of Alcohol and Drug Education*, 56(1), 8–37.

29 Lucidi, F., Grano, C., Leone, L., Lombardo, C. & Pesce, C. (2004). Determinants of the intention to use doping substances. *International Journal of Sport Psychology*, 35, 133–148; Lucidi, F., Zelli, A., Mallia, L., Grano, C., Russo, P. M. & Violani, C. (2008). The social–cognitive mechanisms regulating adolescents' use of doping substances. *Journal of Sports Sciences*, 26(5), 447–456; Zelli, A., Mallia, L. & Lucidi, F. (2010). The contribution of interpersonal appraisals to a social-cognitive analysis of adolescents' doping use. *Psychology of Sport and Exercise*, 11, 204–311.

30 Erickson, K., McKenna, J. & Backhouse, S. H. (2015). A qualitative analysis of the factors that protect athletes against doping in sport. *Psychology of Sport and Exercise*, 16, 149–155.

31 Lenskyi, H. (2003). *Out on the Field: Gender, Sport and Sexualities*. Toronto, ON: Women's Press; White, S., Duda, J. & Keller, M. (1998). The relationship between goal orientation and perceived purposes of sport among youth sport participants, *Journal of Sport Behavior*, 21(4), 474–484.

32 Strean, W. & Holt, N. (2001). Coaches', athletes' and parents' perceptions of fun in youth sports: Assumptions about learning and implications for practice. *Avante*, 63, 1–14.

33 Morris, L., Sallybanks, J., Willis, K. & Makkai, T. (2003). Sport, physical activity and anti-social behaviour in youth. *Trends and Issues in Crime and Criminal Justice, 249,* 1–6.

34 Bairner, A. (2003). Globalization and sport: The nation strikes back. *Phi Kappa Phi Forum, 83*(4), 34–37; Belk, R. (1996). Hyperreality and globalization: Culture in the age of Ronald McDonald. *Journal of International Consumer Marketing, 8*(3), 23–37; Gems, G. (1999). Sports, war, and ideological imperialism. *Peace Review, 11*(4), 573–578; van Bottenburg, M. (2003). Thrown for a loss? (American) football and the European sport space. *The American Behavioral Scientist, 46*(11), 1550–1562.

35 Brissonneau, C. (2006). Deviant careers: The case of cycling, In *Ethics and Social Science Research in Anti-Doping.* WADA Conference, Larnaca, Cyprus, 13–14; Waddington, I. & Smith, A. (2008). *An Introduction to Drugs in Sport: Addicted to Winning.* Oxford, UK: Routledge.

36 Stewart, B. & Smith, A. (2010). Player and athlete attitudes to drugs in Australian sport: implications for policy development. *International Journal of Sport Policy, 2*(1), 65–84.

37 Smith, A. & Stewart, B. (2008). Drug policy in sport: hidden assumptions and inherent contradictions. *Drug and Alcohol Review, 27,* 123–129; Stewart, B. & Smith, A. (2010). Player and athlete attitudes to drugs in Australian sport: implications for policy development. *International Journal of Sport Policy, 2*(1), 65–84.

38 Laure, P. & Binsinger, C. (2005). Adolescent athletes and the demand and supply of drugs to improve performance. *Journal of Sports Science Medicine, 4,* 272–277.

39 Petroczi, A. & Aidman, E. (2008). Psychological drivers in doping: The life-cycle model of performance enhancement. *Substance Abuse Treatment, Prevention, and Policy, 3*(7), 3–12.

40 Stewart, B. & Smith, A. C. T. (2008). Drug use in sport: Implications for public policy. *Journal of Sport and Social Issues, 32*(3), 278–298.

41 European Commission (2014). Study on Doping Prevention. A map of Legal, Regulatory and Prevention Practice Provisions at p. 5.

42 www.theage.com.au/national/schools-urged-to-spell-out-risks-of-sports-drugs-20130517-2js5b.html#ixzz2hjmI5LIv

43 See www.asada.gov.au/education/ for examples of online programs aimed at intervention.

44 www.health.gov.au/internet/main/publishing.nsf/Content/role-of-the-national-integrity-of-sport-unit

45 Victorian Sports Anti-Doping Policy (2012 update at p. 2). Viewed at http://sport.vic.gov.au/file/3226/download?token=yiLdZbbB

46 Bluestone Edge (2013) Access All Levels: Review & scope for a national education program on illicit & performance enhancing drugs for sub-elite & community level sport. Viewed at www.ausport.gov.au/__data/assets/pdf_file/0006/436749/Bluestone_Edge_Access_All_Levels_Report_Oct13_FINAL.pdf

47 www.playbytherules.net.au/

48 www.playbytherules.net.au/resources/videos?pg=3

49 http://play-by-the-rules.s3.amazonaws.com/Resources/R068_Supps_Get_Informed.pdf

50 Access All Levels Report by Bluestone Edge, Recommendation 7 at p. 60.

51 https://elearning.asada.gov.au/

52 www.asada.gov.au/anti-doping-programmes/education/school-lesson-plans

53 www.health.gov.au/internet/main/publishing.nsf/Content/illicit-drugs-in-sport-IDIS-online-education-programme

54 Leeds Beckett Institute for Sport, Physical Activity and Leisure (2015). *Social Psychology of Doping in Sport: A Mixed-Studies Narrative Synthesis prepared for the World Anti-Doping Agency.*

55 To date only 17 studies (Goldberg et al., 1990, 1991, 1996, 2000, 2003, 2007; Grossman & Gieck, 1992; Tricker & Connelly, 1996; Trenhaile et al., 1998; Elliot et al., 2006, 2008; Ranby et al., 2009; Mottram et al., 2008; Laure et al., 2009; James et al., 2010; Jalilian et al., 2011; Nilsson et al., 2004) have evaluated education programmes in relation to behavioural intentions and actions.

56 See www.ohsu.edu/xd/education/schools/school-of-medicine/departments/clinical-departments/medicine/divisions/hpsm/research/atlas-research-findings.cfm and www.ohsu.edu/xd/education/schools/school-of-medicine/departments/clinical-departments/medicine/divisions/hpsm/research/athena-research-findings.cfm

57 Ntoumanis, N., Ng, J. Y., Barkoukis, V. & Backhouse, S. H. (2014). Personal and psychosocial predictors of doping use in physical activity settings: A meta-analysis. *Sports Medicine, 44*(11), 1603–1624.

58 See http://ukad.org.uk

59 Mottram, D, Chester, N. & Gibson, J. (2008). Evaluation of a tutor network system for a national education programme on drug-free sport. *Sport in Society, 11*(5), 560–569.

60 Leeds Beckett Institute for Sport, Physical Activity and Leisure (2015). *Social Psychology of Doping in Sport: A Mixed-Studies Narrative Synthesis prepared for the World Anti-Doping Agency.*

61 Ranby, K. W., Aiken, L. S., Mackinnon, D. P., Elliot, D. L., Moe, E. L., McGinnis, W., & Goldberg, L. (2009). A mediation analysis of the ATHENA intervention for female athletes: prevention of athletic-enhancing substance use and unhealthy weight loss behaviors. *Journal of Pediatric Psychology, 34*(10).

62 Elliot, D. L., Goldberg, L., Moe, E. L., DeFrancesco, C. A., Durham, M. B., McGinnis, W., & Lockwood, C. (2008). Long-term outcomes of the ATHENA (athletes targeting healthy exercise & nutrition alternatives) program for female high school athletes. *Journal of Alcohol and Drug Education, 52*(2).

63 Goldberg, L., Elliot, D. L., MacKinnon, D., Moe, E., Kuehl, K. S., Yoon, M., . . . Williams, J. (2007). Outcomes of a prospective trial of student-athlete drug testing: The Student Athlete Testing Using Random Notification (SATURN) study. *Journal of Adolescent Health, 41*(5), 421–429.

64 Mottram, D, Chester, N & Gibson, J. (2008). Evaluation of a tutor network system for a national education programme on drug-free sport. *Sport in Society, 11*(5), 560–569.

65 James, R., Naughton, D. P. & Petróczi, A. (2010). Promoting functional foods as acceptable alternatives to doping: potential for information-based social marketing approach. *Journal of the International Society of Sports Nutrition, 7*, 37–39.

66 Jalilian, F., Allahverdipour, H., Moeini, B. & Moghimbeigi, A. (2011). Effectiveness of anabolic steroid preventative intervention among gym users: Applying theory of planned behavior. *Health Promotion Perspectives, 1*(1), 32–40.

67 Elbe, A. M. & Brand, R. (2014). The effect of an ethical decision-making training on young athletes' attitudes toward doping. *Ethics & Behavior, 26*(1) 32–44.

68 Laure, P., Favre, A., Binsinger, C. & Mangin, G. (2009). Can self-assertion be targeted in doping prevention actions among adolescent athletes? A randomized controlled trial. *Serbian Journal of Sports Sciences, 3*, 105–110.

69 Leeds Beckett Institute for Sport, Physical Activity and Leisure (2015). *Social Psychology of Doping in Sport: A Mixed-Studies Narrative Synthesis prepared for the World Anti-Doping Agency,* at p. 178.

70 Dunn, M. & White, V. (2011). The epidemiology of anabolic–androgenic steroid use among Australian secondary school students. *The Journal of Science and Medicine in Sport, 14*(1); see also www.abc.net.au/news/2013-07-14/prestigious-high-schools-warn-students-about-drug-use/4818956 and www.theage.com.au/national/sports-drugs-tempt-teens-20131004-2uzvx.html#ixzz2hHuaJiHC

71 For a longer discussion on future research priorities and processes in doping, see Leeds Beckett Institute for Sport, Physical Activity and Leisure (2015). *Social Psychology of Doping in Sport: A Mixed-Studies Narrative Synthesis prepared for the World Anti-Doping Agency.*

5

THOUGHTS, FUNCTIONS, BRAINS AND BOOSTERS

Cognitive enhancers as PIEDS

Introduction

This chapter provides an overview of cognitive enhancement PIEDS, an emerging but nascent subject of interest that promises to grow and gather greater importance. As will be discussed, the area is complex due to the plethora of terms used to describe variants of cognitive enhancers, as well as a variety of overlapping substances that are often labelled as 'smart drugs', including prescription (e.g. methylphenidate, modafinil), non-prescription (e.g., caffeine, gingko biloba, vitamin B6) and illicit (e.g. cocaine, ecstasy) PIEDS. While cognitive enhancement generally refers to the use of drugs or other substances in order to improve cognitive function—typically in relation to brain disorders or dysfunction—the term is employed more specifically in reference to the use of substances by healthy individuals as a form of 'neuro-enhancement'.[1] Cosmetic neurology is another term used to communicate the artificial enhancement of an individual's normal cognitive function.[2] The practice is hotly debated in the neuroscience community, both in relation to its efficacy and, similar to performance enhancing drugs in sport, its ethical implications.

The promise of so-called 'smart drugs' has captured the media's imagination, leading commentators to enthusiastically extol their virtues as almost magical mind enhancers.[3] A quick search of the Internet reveals a proliferation of providers offering a variety of easily available 'brain boosters', along with claims that the substances have been embraced by entrepreneurs, busy executives and college students alike. However, of particular concern to the medical community is the misuse of prescription drugs developed to treat neurodegenerative disorders, such as Alzheimer's and Parkinson's disease, as well as for developmental conditions like attention deficit hyperactivity disorder (ADHD). The consumption of these substances by healthy individuals to enhance alertness, creativity, concentration, memory or problem-solving abilities now occurs within many segments of the population, and is also of interest in the sport and recreation context. In fact, WADA has acknowledged the potential for cognitive enhancing substances to artificially augment athlete ability, and many of the prescription drugs commonly used—or misused—as cognitive enhancers are classified as stimulants and therefore subject to prohibition by WADA during competition.[4]

Common types and use of cognitive enhancers

Cognitive enhancers are popularly referred to as 'nootropics'. The term, meaning 'acting on the mind', which derives from the Greek words *noos* (mind) and *tropein* (towards), was coined in 1972 by Romanian neuroscientist Corneliu Giurgea, after observing the memory-enhancing properties of piracetam in clinical trials.[5] While the term tends to be used interchangeably with 'cognitive enhancer', nootropics originally referred to substances with the following features: enhancement of learning acquisition; resistance to impairing agents; facilitation of inter-hemispheric transfer of information; enhanced resistance to brain 'aggressions'; increased tonic, cortico-subcortical 'control'; and the absence of the usual pharmacological effects of neuro-psychotropic drugs.[6]

The most commonly used prescription drugs for cognitive enhancement include: modafinil, which is used in the treatment of narcolepsy; psychostimulants such as methylphenidate or mixed amphetamine salts including dextroamphetamine, used to treat ADHD; and drugs such as donepezil that are used to treat Alzheimer's disease.[7] The actual usage rate of prescription medications or illicit drugs specifically for the purpose of cognitive enhancement is subject to much debate.[8] One frequently mentioned study, conducted by the scientific journal *Nature*, found that 20% of their readers had used some form of cognitive enhancing drug.[9] However, the results have been widely questioned due to a self-selection sampling method. An Australian study reported that 2.4% of adults surveyed indicated that they had taken prescription medication to enhance concentration or alertness, with 8% declaring that they knew of someone who had done so.[10] While there are many other studies exploring the use of drugs for cognitive enhancement, particularly stimulants, these studies often do not pay any attention to non-medical usage. In fact, while many substances may be used for cognitive enhancement, they may also be consumed for recreational use, such as to provide a feeling of euphoria, to stay awake when studying or even to curb appetite in an effort to lose weight.[11]

Methylphenidate, which is distributed under various trade names, including Ritalin, is reported to be the smart drug of choice for students.[12,13] Many of the studies exploring the non-medical use of prescription drugs for cognitive enhancement have focused on assessing their prevalence in academic contexts. For example, lifetime use of prescription stimulants for cognitive enhancement by high school and university students in Germany was found to be 1.29%,[14] while 7.6% of Swiss university students reported using prescription drugs at least once for cognitive enhancement.[15] In New Zealand, lifetime use amongst university students was found to be 6.6%,[16] and in the United States, non-medical use (although not specifically for cognitive enhancement) of prescription stimulants by high school seniors was reported to be 9.5%,[17] with 16% amongst undergraduate students.[18]

A review of studies highlights a significant variability in the actual prevalence of usage, with lifetime non-medical use of stimulants by students ranging from 1.7 to 55% (the latter in a sample of university students in fraternities).[19] Other research suggests that students are particularly attracted to cognitive enhancers in order to improve learning, reduce nervousness, help with relaxation or sleep and to cope with pressure.[20] However, an alternative explanation for their appeal to students, particularly stimulants, is that they may also impact upon a user's emotional state, which improves engagement with study and its consequent enjoyment.[21]

It remains unclear precisely how cognitive enhancers work, particularly in healthy individuals. However, researchers are making headway into understanding the mechanisms through which some of these enhancers may operate, especially in relation to offsetting cognitive deficits. For example, a recent review proposed 19 different classifications based on the ways various smart drugs may impact on cognition, such as drugs that interact with receptors, drugs that interact with enzymes and drugs that interact with reuptake transporters.[22] Methylphenidate is an example of the latter. It is a stimulant related to amphetamine[23] and acts as a catecholamine reuptake inhibitor;[24] methylphenidate essentially 'increases the synaptic concentrations of dopamine and noradrenaline by blocking their reuptake'.[25] Dopamine has been shown to impact on working memory and also attention.[26]

In contrast, the precise manner in which modafinil operates is not fully understood.[27] However, while the mechanism of action is believed to differ from methylphenidate,[28] it may have similar effects on the reuptake of dopamine and norephinephrine. In addition, the drug may have an effect on neurotransmitters such as serotonin and glutamate.[29]

Nootropics, like racetams, are derivatives of the parent compound piracetam and share a common pyrrolidone structure. Racetams, including piracetam, deliver benefits to impaired patients through positive modulation of glutamate receptors in neurons.[30]

While much of the debate on cognitive enhancement focuses on the use of prescription medication, it should be noted that other non-pharmacological options for augmenting brain power have also elicited interest, resulting in a predictable surge of popularity. 'Brain power' enhancers, including physical exercise, sleep, meditation, yoga, music, computer-based exercises and brain stimulation, can all contribute to maintaining and enhancing optimal cognitive functioning.[31] Furthermore, many of these alternatives are inexpensive, safe and devoid of adverse effects, but they are not nearly as easy as just taking a magic pill.

Impact and ethics of cognitive enhancement

A number of studies have attempted to determine the effectiveness of certain prescription drugs as cognitive enhancers on healthy individuals. In general, research suggests that their effects are modest at best. A systematic review of studies exploring two of the most common drugs used for cognitive enhancement by healthy individuals—methylphenidate and modafinil—found little evidence to support their efficacy.[32] In relation to methylphenidate, the researchers reported that firm conclusions could not be drawn, due to a lack of consistent evidence across studies. However, they recognised some evidence of a positive effect on spatial working memory in healthy individuals. With modafinil, the researchers noted some enhancement, particularly in relation to attention, but no effect was found on memory, mood or motivation.

Some significant challenges when trying to draw conclusions from the limited existing research should be kept in mind. First, there is no consensus as to which battery of tests are best used to assess the effectiveness of cognitive enhancing drugs on healthy individuals in order to enable comparison across studies. Furthermore, very few studies have examined repeated doses or long-term implications of how brain chemistry may be affected,[33] or have tested a range of different dosages.[34] Finally, cognitive enhancers can exhibit both linear and quadratic (U-shaped) effects.[35] This means that an effective dosage facilitating any given cognitive behaviour may also have detrimental (or no) effects on other cognitive behaviours.

In addition to the lack of clarity surrounding the effectiveness of cognitive enhancers, cautions have been issued against the use of prescription drugs, particularly if done so without medical supervision or contrary to their recommended purpose.[36] Some cognitive enhancers carry the potential for serious side effects or addiction, and little is known about the long-term effects of use. Methylphenidate, for example, has been associated with a broad range of potential side effects including headaches, seizures, hypertension, cardiac arrest, anxiety, depression and anaphylactic reactions.[37]

Another area of controversy associated with cognitive-enhancement PIEDS concerns the ethical implications of their use. Similar to PEDS used to artificially augment physical performance, drugs and substances to enhance cognitive performance have attracted ethical questions around whether they constitute cheating, with familiar worries that they compromise a 'level playing field'. For example, some commentary has suggested that the use of cognitive-enhancing drugs reflects a society where high achievers are revered and failure is to be avoided at all costs, irrespective of whether the user is a student, an athlete or a day trader.[38] The acceptance, or the normalisation, of cognitive enhancers has implications for both personal and social identity, as well as the overarching social costs, as these promote a 'hypercompetitive' society as opposed to a more humanitarian one that accepts natural human limitations.[39]

Furthermore, as discussed previously, many athletes practise 'defensive doping' and take PEDS in the belief that their fellow competitors are already users. Similar concerns suggest that increased use and acceptance of cognitive enhancers may lead to coercion—either explicit or implicit—due to the perception that everyone else is taking them.[40,41] Research with German university students confirmed a type of 'contagion effect' whereby students were more willing to use cognitive enhancers if they perceived others in their social circles to be taking them.[42]

Finally, there are also ethical concerns pertaining to the safety of cognitive enhancers, particularly prescription drugs, given the lack of research into the effects on healthy individuals and longer-term usage.[43] However, despite the significant ethical controversy that has been raised around cognitive enhancers, prohibiting their use is likely to fail.[44]

While the efficacy of many of the current means of cognitive enhancement is subject to debate and may only promise modest gains, the future is likely to bring with it more effective products, and increased usage.[45,46] As a result, helpful future research into cognitive enhancement should consider the interaction effects when combined with behavioural approaches to improve cognition, such as on working memory tasks.[47]

Cognitive enhancement in sport

The WADA prohibition of stimulants for in-competition use attempts to capture any substance that may also impact cognition as well as physical performance. As of 2018, this grouping, referred to as 'S6' in the prohibited list,[48] refers to over 60 stimulants, with a catch-all for any 'other substances with a similar chemical structure or similar biological effect(s)'. Methylphenidate appears as a specified substance on the WADA list, while modafinil[49] is non-specified.[50] The distinction between specified and non-specified relates to the amount of discretion associated with imposing a penalty for contravention. Specified substances include more leeway, given an assumption that such substances may be relatively more likely to inadvertently enter an athlete's system.[51]

Recently, modafinil has been carefully monitored as a pharmaceutical, with the European Medicines Agency indicating that while the drug is suitable for treating narcolepsy, it is not recommended for sleep conditions such as obstructive sleep apnoea, shift work sleep disorder and idiopathic hypersomnia,[52] despite such usages being supported in other parts of the world. Nonetheless, the UK Army has reportedly tested a variety of stimulants, including modafinil, aimed at keeping their personnel alert during times of battle, noting that the military is not under the same prohibitions as athletes.[53] The use of modafinil has also been linked in medical studies to astronauts visiting the International Space Station as a means of dealing with disrupted sleep, and in particular, the circadian dyssynchrony brought about by the relatively rapid transitions between light and dark when in orbit.[54] Adoption by institutions renowned for being at the cutting-edge of science is likely to amplify the perception that modafinil has some benefit in increasing memory and alertness, despite its equivocal outcomes as a cognitive enhancer in studies using healthy subjects.[55]

Stimulants that can elicit some sort of cognitive effect on athletes go beyond modafinil and methylphenidate, and can be grouped in a myriad of ways. Docherty,[56] in reviewing the pharmacology of stimulants prohibited by WADA, categorised these by 'mode of action', placing just two substances— meclofenoxate and phenylpiracetam—in the nootropic mode, with the majority of stimulants, including methylphenidate, classified as monoaminomimetic agents. Meclofenoxate, a specified stimulant on the WADA list, is typically used in the treatment of Alzheimer's disease and is said to also aid in recovery from fatigue.[57] Phenylpiracetam, non-specified by WADA, appears largely confined to use in Russia. This drug is an analogue of piracetam, supposedly developed to assist cosmonauts battle fatigue associated with their visits to space stations in the 1980s.[58] It is reported to have anti-amnesic and memory-enhancing effects.[59]

Broadly speaking, the application of nootropics and associated cognitive enhancement remains relatively unexplored for sporting advantages. One website[60] providing information on a range of nootropics, including the 'stacking' of elements for maximum effect, offers an e-book entitled *The Encyclopedia of Nootropics*. The book presents 27 types of nootropics, ranging from natural and dietary supplements (e.g. ginkgo biloba, huperzine A and bacopa monnieri) through to pharmacological stimulants (e.g. adrafinil and modafinil), with 'racetams' (e.g. aniracetam, oxiracetam and pramiracetam) also considered. Racetams, through the activation of glutamate receptors, are purported to aid in memory cognition.[61] While only phenylpiracetam is specifically mentioned on the WADA list, other forms of racetams, given their similar chemical structure, might be of concern to professional athletes.

Challenges for athletes

The uncertainty over the benefits and applications of cognitive enhancers makes it difficult for professional athletes to establish a clear demarcation as to what is permissible and what is not.[62] A saving grace for many athletes would be that stimulants are primarily only banned in competition, and many have a relatively brief half-life, making their evacuation prior to events simple to achieve.[63,64]

To legitimately use cognitive-enhancing substances while in competition requires a Therapeutic Usage Exemption (TUE), a complex and somewhat contentious area in the world of sport given the side effects of some drugs and the need to balance genuine treatment with the potential for unfair enhancement. WADA acknowledges that athletes may have illnesses or conditions that require medications that are on the prohibited list to be used under strict guidelines.[65] To assist, an International Standard for Therapeutic Use Exemptions was created, which details not only the conditions that must be satisfied for a TUE to be granted, but also various application, recognition and confidentiality processes.[66]

Section 4 of the TUE standard is clear on the strict circumstances warranting an exemption: 1) the prohibited substance must be required for the treatment of an 'acute or chronic condition'; 2) for the substance to largely return the athlete to a 'normal state of health' and not 'produce any additional enhancement of performance'; and 3) that there be no reasonable therapeutic alternative. Furthermore, as outlined in Section 5 of the standard, TUE committees include at least three physicians with experience in athlete care and who possess sufficient knowledge of clinical, sports and exercise medicine.

Usage

While the potential benefits of the substances outlined in this chapter may be questionable in terms of pure sporting performance, their usage during training periods might be advantageous given their ease of availability, and potential to enhance not just physical elements such as recovery, but the many complex and taxing mental tasks that athletes perform regularly. These may include many hours of performance or game analysis, pre-performance anxiety, tactical preparation and increased travel interrupting sleep patterns.

While studies on the use of cognitive enhancers in sport are not yet available, some informative data can be assembled, including the numbers of athletes suffering from conditions for which stimulants are a recommended form of treatment. For example, Major League Baseball (MLB) in the US, which has endured allegations of substance abuse by leading players in the past, is now more proactive in regulating and monitoring players.[67] As a result, the MLB produces an annual report that summarises their drug-testing regimen. In 2016, this report[68] detailed 8281 tests conducted during the reporting period, including 6634 urine samples and 1647 blood samples. These tests yielded 15 adverse findings, three of which were for stimulant use.

MLB is played across a season where athletes compete on a highly frequent basis,[69] making the ability to manage permissible substance use in and out of competition extremely difficult. Interestingly, the report notes that 107 TUEs were granted during the period, 105 of which were for attention deficit disorder. That places the proportion of players in MLB seeking a therapeutic exemption for attention deficit disorder at approximately 7.5%.[70] Comparing that to the general adult US population is challenging, as attention deficit disorder tracking mainly focuses on children, despite the fact that it does also affect older groups. Nevertheless, a 2006 report[71] estimated the prevalence of adult ADHD in the United States to be 4.4%, although substantial increases in childhood diagnosis in recent years are likely to have raised that number.[72] It should also be noted that the prevalence of this condition is skewed strongly towards males.[73] Further, as exercise benefits many children and adults with ADHD,[74] it is possible that sufferers may be drawn to competitive sport as a way of dealing with the condition.[75]

While not technically considered a cognitive enhancer, the addition of the relatively unknown drug meldonium (an anti-ischaemia medication with limited distribution, primarily in Eastern Europe) to the WADA banned list on 1 January 2016, provides some insight into how athletes might behave with regards to prescription medications. Meldonium is classed as an S4 metabolic modulator,[76] making it non-permissible at all times. According to a tweet[77] by WADA in mid-April in 2016, testing had revealed 172 adverse analytical findings (positive tests) in just 104 days of the substance moving onto the banned list. While the number of athletes testing positive perhaps speaks more directly to the dissemination of information on which substances have been added to the WADA list, it does raise some questions as to how many professional athletes were in need of the medication at the time it was legal. After all, it could be reasonably expected that far more stopped usage (or sought an exemption) once the ban came into force.

A natural inclination for athletes to consider using drugs and substances not on the WADA list is to be expected, given the range of competitive and commercial factors that weigh heavily on their performance expectations. Legal drugs or substances that can offer some performance benefit, even if their therapeutic need is questionable, can be appealing to many in the search for a winning edge. Most serious athletes are likely to be on vitamin and other (legal) substance regimens for much of their lives in what has been described as akin to an '. . . arms-race quality to performance enhancing strategies in sport'.[78]

Implications and issues

If we accept that sporting endeavours demand considerable preparation and not just execution, how athletes train their bodies and minds must be critical in the lead-up to high performance. Cognitive enhancers that facilitate greater learning and memory capability should be invaluable in almost every sport given the complexities of performance execution through technical analysis, enhanced coaching and kinesiology. Elite athletes must make numerous micro-decisions under intense pressure and, for the most part, are trained to revert to their 'muscle-memory'.

The role of nootropics and cognitive enhancers in this process raises enormously complex ethical issues that can be applied more broadly to society, as previously highlighted. While pharmacological interventions to return individuals to a normal base of operation, or limit cognitive decline, are socially and culturally accepted, the provision for cognitive enrichment of otherwise healthy (and indeed in the case of sport, typically physically elite) individuals remains decidedly ambiguous.

Uncertainty over the ethics of cognitive enhancement may be due partly to sport's long history as a physical endeavour. That is, sport has always largely revolved around physical exertion: running, jumping, lifting, throwing, swimming, kicking and so forth. While cerebral decision making has always featured, its importance has recently been elevated given the increasing data and related information provided to modern athletes. To take just one example, professional tennis players, once adept at sizing up the strengths and weaknesses of opponents and matching their physical exploits based on this assessment, now have access to data on every conceivable permutation and combination in a match. While some sports assist athletes in information management—photography of formations, headsets in helmets and complex play-charts all feature in American Football, for example—a tennis player is 'on his or her own' in a professional match, technically forbidden from communicating with coaches or using technological aids.

The trickle-down effect on amateur and recreational athletes in the area of cognitive enhancement is likely to be significant. Given their popular perception as smart drugs, the use of terminology such as nootropics suggests that favourable brain training is possible. Indeed, the general appearance of cognitive enhancers in society in the context of improved study or child learning has the potential to become normalised. As a result, the ethical question of using cognitive enhancement more broadly in society is often equated to doping in sport.[79] Research has indicated that adults are twice as likely to accept the use of cognitive enhancers compared to performance enhancing drugs (i.e. doping) use by athletes,[80] although levels of acceptance in both cases still remain low.

With society adept at 'popping a pill' to solve ailments, cognitive enhancers in a portable and easily ingestible form makes them far easier to justify for the recreational sportsperson looking to overcome the fatigue of a workday before playing in a local club competition. Consumption may be further rationalised given the perceptions (if not the reality) of many nootropic and cognitive-enhancement agents as being relatively benign in terms of side effects. This situation may already have manifested, with a study of recreational triathletes in Germany suggesting that as many as 15% of participants were engaged in cognitive enhancement through substances such as modafinil and methylphenidate. Interestingly, 13% of the same participants indicated usage of drugs like steroids, EPO or growth hormones, lending credibility to the theory that significant cross-over exists between body and brain-doping.[81]

The effects that substances such as modafinil and methylphenidate have on athletes are not well understood, but some insights are beginning to appear in other competitive contexts. In a widely reported study published in early 2017,[82] European researchers found cognitive improvements in highly skilled chess players who used nootropics as well as mega-doses of caffeine, suggesting that even high-functioning thinkers can yield benefits from cognitive enhancement. Caffeine has the advantage that it only appears on WADA's monitoring programme, and has not been explicitly prohibited since 2004.

The findings of the chess study are particularly interesting for understanding the complexity of cognitive enhancement through the use of stimulants. While one would presume that a stimulant, given its name, would speed up the thinking process or increase the quality of thinking in a given time period, the results suggest this only partially occurs. In fact, high-level chess players spent more time on each decision, making calculations and assessments that were both more thorough and more time consuming. In effect, better decisions were made, but were made more slowly. The 'increased reflection time' reported by the study was calculated at approximately two minutes more per match[83] (chess players had 15 minutes per match for their moves) for those using the stimulants. As some chess is played to a time limit, some players in the study fell foul of standard time regulations, but the overall quality of play could be improved if the effect of time regulations were excluded.

The implications, if applied to sport more broadly, are fascinating if cognitive enhancers prioritise reflection-based decision making rather than the speed of decision making. Chess constitutes a focused cognitive pursuit and requires a succession of mentally challenging matches, the implication being that generalisability to sport might be limited. At the very least, more research remains essential. However, the time 'trade-off', in principle, poses an interesting conundrum if applied more broadly, given that sport is often played under the intense pressure of the kind of rapid-fire decision making that can distinguish the amateur from the professional. Such a distinction may be the difference between life and death for a racing car driver. Or, it might compromise an NFL quarterback who takes more sacks because of increased processing time, but provides him with a greater proportion of successful passes when sacks are avoided, leading to an awkward counterbalance between positive and negative effects. Each sport and each situation will have its own nuances, making the impact of cognitive enhancement difficult to categorise. It is also worth noting that the concept of a speed–accuracy trade-off has been explored with differing results by other researchers, albeit outside of sport.[84]

The impact of caffeine adds further weight to the role it plays in performance enhancement. Caffeine seemingly has the dual role of boosting physical performance by limiting perceptions of fatigue,[85] and mental performance through increased processing time,[86] giving it an unassailable claim to being the world's most popular performance enhancing drug.[87]

Conclusion

The focus of cognitive enhancement research on improved memory, learning and task fulfilment has meant that the impact in more physical pursuits such as sport has not yet been fully explored. WADA only bans stimulants during in-competition activities, leaving fertile training periods where elite athletes can pursue cognitive enhancement. At the very least, a caffeine regimen would be given consideration by most athletes as it is not on the banned list of stimulants. Numerous ethical issues remain, however, particularly in the use of prescription drugs for the cognitive enhancement of healthy adults or through therapeutic use exemptions in elite sport. While cognitive enhancers may at best offer modest improvements in memory or decision making, there remains a need for significant contextual research to better understand the mechanisms of these improvements, mainly in terms of speed and accuracy trade-offs, and the potential for increased reflection time leading to deeper thinking. With athletes already likely to be relatively attuned to the decision processes of their sports, the potential for cognitive enhancers to interfere with behaviours or other cognitive processes in a negative way cannot be discounted. For the recreational athlete, there appears to be limited evidence to suggest that cognitive enhancement is a significant issue. However, its relative acceptance in comparison to strength or endurance doping is an area of concern, suggesting that policies will be needed to ensure that 'brain-doping' does not become a social norm on playing fields across the world.

Notes

1 Frati, P., Kyriakou, C., Del Rio, A., Marinelli, E., Vergallo, G. M., Zami, S. & Busardò, F. P. (2015). Smart drugs and synthetic androgens for cognitive and physical enhancement: Revolving doors of cosmetic neurology. *Current Neuropharmacology*, *13*(1), 5–11.
2 Chatterjee, A. (2007). Cosmetic neurology and cosmetic surgery: Parallels, predictions, and challenges. *Cambridge Quarterly of Healthcare Ethics*, *16*, 129–137.

3 Partridge, B. J., Bell, S. K., Lucke, J. C., Yeates, S., & Hall, W. D. (2011). Smart drugs as "common as coffee": Media hype about neuroenhancement. *PLoS One, 6*(11), e28416. doi:10.1371/journal.pone.0028416

4 www.wada-ama.org/en/prohibited-list/prohibited-in-competition/stimulants, accessed 24 November, 2017.

5 Froestl, W., Muhs, A. & Pfeifer, A. (2012). Cognitive enhancers (nootropics). Part 1: Drugs interacting with receptors. *Journal of Alzheimer's Disease, 32*, 793–887.

6 Giurgea, C. & Salama, B. (1977). Nootropic drugs, *Progress in Neuro-Psychopharmocology, 1*(3/4), 235–247.

7 Partridge, B. J., Bell, S. K., Lucke, J. C., Yeates, S. & Hall, W. D. (2011). Smart drugs as "common as coffee": Media hype about neuroenhancement. *PLoS One, 6*(11), e28416. doi:10.1371/journal.pone.0028416

8 Smith, M. E. & Farah, M. J. (2011). Are prescription stimulants "smart pills"?: The epidemiology and cognitive neuroscience of prescription stimulant use by normal healthy individuals. *Psychological Bulletin, 137*(5), 717–741.

9 Maher, B. (2008). Poll results: Look who's doping. *Nature, 452*, 674–675.

10 Partridge, B., Lucke, J. & Hall, W. (2012). A comparison of attitudes toward cognitive enhancement and legalized doping in sport in a community sample of Australian adults. *AJOB Primary Research, 3*(4) 81–86.

11 Smith, M. E. & Farah, M. J. (2011). Are prescription stimulants "smart pills"?: The epidemiology and cognitive neuroscience of prescription stimulant use by normal healthy individuals. *Psychological Bulletin, 137*(5), 717–741.

12 Franke, A. G., Bonertz, C., Christmann, M., Huss, M., Fellgiebel, A. Hildt, E. & Lieb, K. (2010). Non-medical use of prescription stimulants and illicit use of stimulants for cognitive enhancement in pupils and students in Germany. *Pharmacopsychiatry, 44*, 60–66.

13 Maier, L. J., Liechti, M. E. & Schaub, M. P. (2013). To dope of not to dope: Neuroenhancment with prescription drugs and drugs of abuse among Swiss university students. *PLoS One, 8*(11): e77967. https://doi.org/10.1371/journalpone.0077967

14 Franke, A. G., Bonertz, C., Christmann, M., Huss, M., Fellgiebel, A. Hildt, E. & Lieb, K. (2010). Non-medical use of prescription stimulants and illicit use of stimulants for cognitive enhancement in pupils and students in Germany. *Pharmacopsychiatry, 44*, 60–66.

15 Maier, L. J., Liechti, M. E. & Schaub, M. P. (2013). To dope of not to dope: Neuroenhancment with prescription drugs and drugs of abuse among Swiss university students. *PLoS One, 8*(11): e77967. https://doi.org/10.1371/journalpone.0077967

16 Ram, S., Hussainy, S., Henning, M., Jensen, M. & Russell, B. (2016). Prevalence of cognitive enhancer use among New Zealand tertiary students. *Drug and Alcohol Review, 35*, 345–351.

17 McCabe, S. E. & West, B. T. (2013). Medical and nonmedical use of prescription stimulants: Results from a national multicohort study. *Journal of the American Academy of Child and Adolescent Psychiatry, 52*(12), 1272–1280.

18 Prudhomme White, B., Becker-Blease, K. A. & Grace-Bishop, K. (2006). Stimulant medication use, misuse, and abuse in an undergraduate and graduate student sample. *Journal of American College Health, 54*(5), 261–268.

19 Smith, M. E. & Farah, M. J. (2011). Are prescription stimulants "smart pills"?: The epidemiology and cognitive neuroscience of prescription stimulant use by normal healthy individuals. *Psychological Bulletin, 137*(5), 717–741.

20 Maier, L. J., Liechti, M. E. & Schaub, M. P. (2013). To dope of not to dope: Neuroenhancment with prescription drugs and drugs of abuse among Swiss university students. *PLoS One, 8*(11): e77967. https://doi.org/10.1371/journalpone.0077967

21 Vrecko, S. (2013). Just how cognitive is "cognitive enhancement"? On the significance of emotions in university students' experiences with study drugs. *AJOB Neuroscience, 4*(1), 4–12. DOI: 10.1080/21507740.2012.740141

22 Froestl, W., Muhs, A. & Pfeifer, A. (2012). Cognitive enhancers (nootropics). Part 1: Drugs interacting with receptors. *Journal of Alzheimer's Disease, 32*, 793–887.

23 De Jonge, R., Bolt, I., Schermer, M. & Olivier, B. (2008). Botox for the brain: Enhancement of cognition, mood and pro-social behavior and blunting of unwanted memories. *Neuroscience and Biobehavioral Reviews*, 32, 760–776.

24 Franke, A. G. Gransmark, P. Agricola, A., Schuhle, K., Rommel, T., Sebastian, A., Ballo H. E., Gorbulev, S., Gerdes, C., Frank, B., Ruckes, C., Tuscher, O. & Lieb, K. (2017). Methylphenidate, modafinil, and caffeine for cognitive enhancement in chess: A double-blind, randomised controlled trial. *European Neuropsychopharmacology, 27*(3) 248–260. http://dx.doi.org/10.1016/j.euroneuro.2017.01.006

25 de Jonge, R., Bolt, I., Schermer, M. & Olivier, B. (2008). Botox for the brain: Enhancement of cognition, mood and pro-social behavior and blunting of unwanted memories. *Neuroscience and Biobehavioral Reviews, 32*, 760–776.

26 Husain, M. & Mehta, M. A. (2011). Cognitive enhancement by drugs in health and disease. *Trends in Cognitive Science, 15*(1), 28–36.

27 de Jonge, R., Bolt, I., Schermer, M. & Olivier, B. (2008). Botox for the brain: Enhancement of cognition, mood and pro-social behavior and blunting of unwanted memories. *Neuroscience and Biobehavioral Reviews, 32*, 760–776.

28 Repantis, D., Schlattmann, P., Laisney, O. & Heuser, I. (2010). Modafinil and methylphenidate for neuroenhancment in healthy individuals: A systematic review. *Pharmacological Research, 62*, 187–206.

29 Franke, A. G., Gransmark, P., Agricola, A., Schuhle, K., Rommel, T., Sebastian, A., Ballo H. E., Gorbulev, S., Gerdes, C., Frank, B., Ruckes, C., Tuscher, O. & Lieb, K. (2017). Methylphenidate, modafinil, and caffeine for cognitive enhancement in chess: A double-blind, randomised controlled trial. *European Neuropsychopharmacology, 27*(3), 248–260. http://dx.doi.org/10.1016/j.euroneuro.2017.01.006

30 Copani, A., Genazzani, A. A., Aleppo, G., Casabona, G., Canonico, P. L., Scapagnini, U. & Nicoletti, F. (1992). Nootropic drugs positively modulate α-amino-3-hydroxy-5-methyl-4-isoxazolepropionic acid-sensitive glutamate receptors in neuronal cultures. *Journal of Neurochemistry, 58*, 1199–1204.

31 Sachdeva, A., Kumar, K. & Singh Anand, K. (2015). Non-pharmacological cognitive enhancers: Current perspectives. *Journal of Clinical and Diagnostic Research, 9*(7), 1–6.

32 Repantis, D., Schlattmann, P., Laisney, O. & Heuser, I. (2010). Modafinil and methylphenidate for neuroenhancment in healthy individuals: A systematic review. *Pharmacological Research, 62*, 187–206.

33 Husain, M. & Mehta, M. A. (2011). Cognitive enhancement by drugs in health and disease. *Trends in Cognitive Science, 15*(1), 28–36.

34 Repantis, D., Schlattmann, P., Laisney, O. & Heuser, I. (2010). Modafinil and methylphenidate for neuroenhancment in healthy individuals: A systematic review. *Pharmacological Research, 62*, 187–206.

35 de Jonge, R., Bolt, I., Schermer, M. & Olivier, B. (2008). Botox for the brain: Enhancement of cognition, mood and pro-social behavior and blunting of unwanted memories. *Neuroscience and Biobehavioral Reviews, 32*, 760–776.

36 Cleveland, E. (2016). What's missing from the current smart drugs debate? *Society, 53*(3), 237–239.

37 Frati, P., Kyriakou, C., Del Rio, A., Marinelli, E., Vergallo, G. M., Zami, S. & Busardò, F. P. (2015). Smart drugs and synthetic androgens for cognitive and physical enhancement: Revolving doors of cosmetic neurology. *Current Neuropharmacology, 13*(1), 5–11.

38 Cleveland, E. (2016). What's missing from the current smart drugs debate? *Society, 53*(3), 237–239.

39 Wagner, N.-F., Robinson, J. & Weibking, C. (2015). The ethics of neuroenhancement: Smart drugs, competition and society. *International Journal of Technoethics, 6*(1), 10–20.

40 Cleveland, E. (2016). What's missing from the current smart drugs debate? *Society, 53*(3), 237–239.

41 Farah, M. J., Illes, J., Cook-Deegan, R., Gardner, H., Kandel, E., King, P., Parens, E., Sakakian, B. & Wolpe, P. R. (2004). Neurocognitive enhancement: What can we do and what should we do? *Nature Reviews Neuroscience, 5*, 421–425.

42 Sattler, S., Forlini, C., Racine, E. & Sauer, C. (2013). Impact of contextual factors and substance characteristics on perspectives toward cognitive enhancement. *PLoS One*, *8*(8), e71452. doi:10.1371/journal.pone.0071452

43 Cakic, V. (2009). Smart drugs for cognitive enhancement: Ethical and pragmatic considerations in the era of cosmetic neurology. *Journal of Medical Ethics*, *35*, 611–615.

44 Cakic, V. (2009). Smart drugs for cognitive enhancement. Ethical and pragmatic considerations in the era of cosmetic neurology. *Journal of Medical Ethics*, *35*, 611–615.

45 Cakic, V. (2009). Smart drugs for cognitive enhancement: Ethical and pragmatic considerations in the era of cosmetic neurology. *Journal of Medical Ethics*, *35*, 611–615.

46 Farah, M. J., Illes, J., Cook-Deegan, R., Gardner, H., Kandel, E., King, P., Parens, E., Sakakian, B. & Wolpe, P. R. (2004). Neurocognitive enhancement: What can we do and what should we do? *Nature Reviews Neuroscience*, *5*, 421–425.

47 Husain, M. & Mehta, M. A. (2011). Cognitive enhancement by drugs in health and disease. *Trends in Cognitive Science*, *15*(1), 28–36.

48 www.wada-ama.org/sites/default/files/prohibited_list_2018_en.pdf, accessed 6 December, 2017.

49 Adrafanil, a prodrug to modafinil (metabolised *in vivo* to modafinil) is also listed; despite being discontinued in 2011, it is reported as still being available off-label in North America (see www.braintropic.com/nootropics/adrafinil/).

50 Under the WADA Code, an athlete can face a ban of up to two years if a Specified Substance is present in their sample. They could face a maximum of four years for a Non-Specified Substance.

51 www.wada-ama.org/en/questions-answers/prohibited-list#item-387, accessed 6 December, 2017.

52 www.ema.europa.eu/docs/en_GB/document_library/Referrals_document/Modafinil_31/WC500099177.pdf, accessed 5 December, 2017.

53 See http://news.bbc.co.uk/2/hi/uk_news/politics/6083840.stm, accessed 25 November, 2017.

54 Thirsk, R., Kuipers, A., Mukai, C. & Williams, D. (2009). The space-flight environment: the International Space Station and beyond. *CMAJ*, *180*(12), 1216–1220.

55 Repantis, D., Schlattmann, P., Laisney, O. & Heuser, I. (2010). Modafinil and methylphenidate for neuroenhancment in healthy individuals: A systematic review. *Pharmacological Research*, *62*, 187–206.

56 Docherty, J. R. (2008). Pharmacology of stimulants prohibited by the World Anti-Doping Agency (WADA). *British Journal of Pharmacology*, *154*, 606–622.

57 Haavisto, M. (2011). Reviving the Broken Marionette: Treatments for CFS/ME and Fibromyalgia. Self-published.

58 https://medi.ru/info/427, accessed 23 November, 2017.

59 Malykh, A. G. & Sadaie, M. R. (2010) Piracetam and piracetam-like drugs from Basic science to novel clinical applications to CNS disorders. *Drugs*, *70*(3), 287–312.

60 www.braintropic.com.

61 Copani, A., Genazzani, A. A., Aleppo, G., Casabona, G., Canonico, P. L., Scapagnini, U. & Nicoletti, F. (1992). Nootropic drugs positively modulate alpha-amino-3-hydroxy-5-methyl-4-isoxazolepropionic acid-sensitive glutamate receptors in neuronal cultures. *Journal of Neurochemistry*, *58*(4), 1199–1204.

62 Docherty, J. R. (2008). Pharmacology of stimulants prohibited by the World Anti-Doping Agency (WADA). *British Journal of Pharmacology*, *154*, 606–622.

63 www.nuvigil.com/PDF/Full_Prescribing_Information.pdf

64 Kimko, H. C., Cross, J. T. 7 Abernethy, D. R. (1999). Pharmacokinetics and clinical effectiveness of methylphenidate. *Clinical Pharmacokinetics*, *37*(6), 457–470.

65 www.wada-ama.org/en/what-we-do/science-medical/therapeutic-use-exemptions, accessed 28 November, 2017.

66 www.wada-ama.org/sites/default/files/resources/files/WADA-2015-ISTUE-Final-EN.pdf, accessed 28 November, 2017.

67 www.theguardian.com/sport/2013/aug/02/biogenesis-PEDS-scandal-explained, accessed 28 November, 2017.

68 www.mlbplayers.com/ViewArticle.dbml?DB_OEM_ID=34000&ATCLID=211336296, accessed 26 November, 2017.

69 Teams in MLB play 162 games per season, spread across approximately six months.

70 In discussing the issue of MLB Therapeutic Use Exemptions, Lakhan & Kirchgessner (2012) noted at the time that 7.6% of the 1354 players on major-league rosters have been diagnosed with ADHD. See Lakhan, A. E. & Kirchgessner, A. (2012). Prescription stimulants in individuals with and without attention deficit hyperactivity disorder: misuse, cognitive impact, and adverse effects. *Brain and Behavior, 2*(5) 661–677.

71 www.ncbi.nlm.nih.gov/pubmed/16585449, accessed 24 November, 2017.

72 www.additudemag.com/the-statistics-of-adhd/, accessed 28 November, 2017.

73 Visser, S. N., Danielson, M. L., Bitsko, R. H., Holbrook, J. R., Kogan Ghandour, R. M., Perou, R. & Blumberg, S. J. (2014). Trends in the Parent-Report of Health Care Provider-Diagnosed and Medicated Attention-Deficit/Hyperactivity Disorder: United States, 2003–2011. *Journal of the American Academy of Child & Adolescent Psychiatry, 53*(1), 34–46.

74 White, R. D., Harris, G. D. & Gibson, M. E. (2013). Attention deficit hyperactivity disorder and athletes. *Sports Health, 6*(2), 149–156.

75 Conant-Norville, D. O. & Tofler, I. R. (2005). Attention deficit/hyperactivity disorder and psychopharmacologic treatments in the athlete. *Clinical Sports Medicine, 24*, 829–843.

76 www.wada-ama.org/en/prohibited-list/prohibited-at-all-times/hormone-and-metabolic-modulators, accessed 27 November, 2017.

77 https://twitter.com/wada_ama/status/720250814246346752, accessed 28 November, 2017.

78 Thompson, H. (2012). Performance enhancement: Superhuman athletes. *Nature, 487*, 287–289.

79 Cakic, V. (2009). Smart drugs for cognitive enhancement: Ethical and pragmatic considerations in the era of cosmetic neurology. *Journal of Medical Ethics, 35*, 611–615.

80 Partridge, B., Lucke, J. & Hall, W. (2012). A comparison of attitudes toward cognitive enhancement and legalized doping in sport in a community sample of Australian adults. *AJOB Primary Research, 3*(4), 81–86.

81 Dietz, P., Ulrich, R., Dalaker, R., Streigel, H., Franke, A. G., Lieb, K. & Perikles, S. (2013). Associations between physical and cogntive doping—a cross-sectional study in 2,997 triathletes. *PLOS One, 8*(11), e78702 doi:10.1371/journal.pone.0078702

82 Franke, A. G., Gransmark, P., Agricola, A., Schuhle, K., Rommel, T., Sebastian, A., Ballo H. E., Gorbulev, S., Gerdes, C., Frank, B., Ruckes, C., Tuscher, O. & Lieb, K. (2017). Methylphenidate, modafinil, and caffeine for cognitive enhancement in chess: A double-blind, randomised controlled trial. *European Neuropsychopharmacology, 27*(3), 248–260.

83 The average reflection (thinking) time per 15-minute game for participants reported in the Franke et al. (2017) study was 436.8 seconds on placebo, 552.8 seconds with modafinil, 547.3 with methylphenidate and 530.1 with caffeine.

84 See Winder-Rhodes, S., Chamberlain, S., Idris, M., Robbins, T., Sahakian, B. & Muller, U. (2010). Effects of modafinil and prazosin on cognitive and physiological functions in healthy volunteers. *Journal of Psychopharmacology, 24*(11), 1649–1657.

85 www.sportsdietitians.com.au/factsheets/supplements/caffeine/, accessed 24 November, 2017.

86 Franke, A. G., Gransmark, P., Agricola, A., Schuhle, K., Rommel, T., Sebastian, A., Ballo H. E., Gorbulev, S., Gerdes, C., Frank, B., Ruckes, C., Tuscher, O. & Lieb, K. (2017). Methylphenidate, modafinil, and caffeine for cognitive enhancement in chess: A double-blind, randomised controlled trial, *European Neuropsychopharmacology, 27*(3), 248–260.

87 www.theatlantic.com/health/archive/2014/03/how-athletes-strategically-use-caffeine/283758/, accessed 30 November, 2017.

6

PROTEIN, PROHORMONES, STEROIDS AND STIMULANTS

Performance and image enhancing drugs and substances typology of classes

Introduction

In this chapter, we provide a detailed PIEDS typology consisting of 15 classes. Any attempt to typologise PIEDS must navigate the complexity of types, effects and compounds. For example, many different forms of PIEDS can be employed to target similar physical outcomes, but each may comprise a completely different effect size and risk profile. As previously highlighted, in order to account for the significant differences between PIEDS, we have classified them across three main strata, Dietary and Nutritional Supplements (DNS); Enhancement and Augmentation (EA); and Performance Enhancing Drugs (PEDS).

DNS have been further sub-categorised into four types of effects: 1) Power & Muscle; 2) Energy & Endurance; 3) Fat & Metabolism; and 4) Immunity & Inflammation. EA comprises a single category, labelled number '5'. PEDS encompasses 10 sub-categories, from '6–15': 6) Anabolic Agents; 7) Hormones; 8) Hormone Manipulators; 9) Beta-2 Agonists; 10) Masking Agents; 11) Stimulants (and 11b Cognitive Enhancers); 12) Pain & Pleasure Narcotics; 13) Adrenal Manipulators; 14) Psychoactives; and 15) Anti-inflammatories.

Our classification decisions also straddle a diverse range of legal, illicit, banned and permitted compounds, some useless, some innocuous, some mildly helpful, some advantageous, some potent and some dangerous. It is therefore problematic to place a mild dietary and nutritional supplement in the same classification schema as a powerful pharmaceutical. In addition, we favoured a classification system consistent with conventional and well-accepted groupings. To that end, where possible, we have maintained a classification schema for PEDS consistent with WADA's model. A summary matrix is provided next for each sub-category of PIEDS, which highlights each category's major descriptors.

Summary matrix

Category	Harm profile	Legal status/ WADA status	Performance effects	Performance magnitude	User profile
A. DNS					
Power & muscle	None to mild	Legal Permitted	Size Strength Recovery	None to small	Bodybuilders Athletes Image users
Energy & endurance			Longer efforts Less fatigue		Athletes Students Shift workers
Fat & metabolism			Burns calories Fat loss		Image users Weight-class athletes
Immunity & inflammation			Recovery Health		Athletes Heath users
B. EA					
Enhancement/ augmentation	Moderate	Legal (under medical supervision) Permitted	None to negative	N/A	Image users Bodybuilders
C. PEDS					
Anabolic agents	Moderate to significant	Mostly illegal Mostly banned (subject to therapeutic use exemptions)	Size Strength Recovery Fat loss	Medium to very strong	Athletes Bodybuilders Fitness users Image users
Hormones			Size Strength		Bodybuilders Athletes
Hormone manipulators			Size Strength		Bodybuilders Athletes
Beta-2 agonists			Size Aerobic performance Fat loss		Bodybuilders Fitness competitors
Masking agents			Conceals PEDS		Competitive athletes
Stimulants			Concentration Less fatigue Fat loss		Athletes Weight loss users Fitness competitors Recreational users
Pain/pleasure narcotics			Recovery Relaxation Injury return		Athletes Pleasure seekers
Adrenal manipulators			Steady hands Concentration Relaxation Recovery		Controlled skill sport players Recreational relaxation-seekers
Psychoactives			Stress release Relaxation		Elite athletes Pleasure seekers
Anti-inflammatories			Pain relief Injury return		Serious athletes

CATEGORY 1. *Power and muscle DNS*	Protein supplements (and weight gainers) Amino acids Muscle builders Testosterone boosters
Supplement	*Summary of effects*
Protein supplements and weight gainers: Whey protein Milk protein Casein protein Beef protein Soy protein Hemp protein Rice protein Pea protein	Protein supplements—usually in the form of flavoured powder concentrates and isolates—are consumed orally in order to add dietary protein, especially during 'peri-workout' periods (before, during and/or after exercise). The powders may be derived from a range of sources including milk (most common in the forms of whey and casein), rice, pea, hemp, beef and fish. Supplemental protein works by enhancing muscle protein synthesis, especially following intense muscular exercise, thereby bolstering recovery and facilitating muscular hypertrophy (growth).[1] With longer, more frequent and heavier volumes of training, protein supplementation promotes muscle size and strength in both untrained and trained individuals, which means that it has benefits for almost everyone from the novice recreational exerciser to the elite weightlifter. Some evidence suggests that protein supplementation accelerates aerobic endurance as well as anaerobic power.[2] For these reasons, protein supplements are the most common DNS amongst athletes and appearance-oriented users interested in larger muscles. Protein supplementation has also been shown to preserve muscle mass in older adults, as well as during caloric restriction.[3] As a result, protein powders are increasing in popularity with heath-conscious older exercisers and middle-aged dieters. Numerous studies have demonstrated that the effects of protein supplementation are similar across all protein classes.[4] For example, whey and rice protein isolate after exercise have been shown to improve body composition and physical performance.[5] In addition, protein supplementation at other times, such as prior to sleep, has been linked to superior muscular recovery and hypertrophy.[6] While using protein supplements consistently delivers acute effects on muscular anabolism, their effects remain debated. Clinical studies have recorded effects ranging from the negligible and marginal, to the mild and moderate.[7] It is certainly clear that the promises of 'massive gains' plastered on protein labels and print and electronic promotions do not match the

Supplement	Summary of effects
	results of controlled trials. There is no evidence that protein supplementation is more effective than food protein sources.[8] Protein supplements are generally regarded as safe and convenient, if not always necessary.[9] In fact, whey protein has been associated with a lower risk of metabolic disorders and cardiovascular diseases.[10] Prospective users with dysfunctional livers or kidneys should seek advice from a medical practitioner prior to consuming protein supplements.
Amino acids Branched-chain amino acids Essential amino acids Histidine Isoleucine Leucine Lysine Methionine Phenylalanine Threonine Tryptophan Valine	Protein contains amino acids, of which 20 are considered biologically significant and nine are essential to a complete nutritional profile.[11] If ingested individually, various amino acids are associated with improved physical health and athletic performance. As a result, amino acids are placed amongst the top five most popular sports supplements.[12] For the athlete or appearance-conscious individual, taking certain amino acids may strengthen the metabolic transformations necessary to induce muscle growth, endurance, recovery and fat loss.[13] Amino acids can be found in any protein source. Several of the most popular amino acids are reviewed in forthcoming sections, as they each putatively deliver different physical effects. Under the Power and Muscle category, the most prominent amino acid DNS comprises a combination of three—branched-chain amino acids (BCAA)—that have been associated with the processes of muscular growth and recovery.[14] BCAAs refer to three amino acids: leucine, isoleucine and valine. BCAA supplementation has been shown to elevate muscle protein synthesis and enhance muscle growth over time.[15] It also prevents fatigue and supports recovery after intense exercise.[16] However, the evidence suggests that additional supplementation is unnecessary for people with an adequate protein intake.[17]
Creatine monohydrate	Creatine monohydrate is a molecule produced in the body that releases energy to aid cellular function. Creatine supplementation therefore aids the brain, bones, muscles and liver. The benefits of creatine include improvements in lean mass,[18] power[19] and muscle size.[20] Creatine is safe, although excessive dosages have been linked to digestive discomfort.[21]

Supplement	Summary of effects
Testosterone boosters: D-Aspartic acid Horny goat weed Maca *Tribulus terrestris* Longifolia Jack Ecdysteroids Fenugreek Holy basil Stinging nettle *Coleus forskohlii* Ginger Saw palmetto Vitamin D	Testosterone boosters purportedly increase testosterone levels in the blood. Higher testosterone is associated with muscle growth. As the corresponding list confirms, the number of supplements claiming to boost testosterone is too large to review individually. However, studies investigating testosterone boosters suggest that they do not work. Most testosterone boosters have no clinical effect,[22] while the handful that do so appear to deliver marginal benefits unless the user suffers from a deficiency in an essential area, such as vitamin D.[23] Also problematic is that many supplement brands report the effects from studies conducted on rodents rather than human trials.[24] Some of the more popular testosterone boosters include vitamin D and curcumin. These are reviewed later as 'antioxidants', but can have a mild testosterone-boosting effect. Others demonstrating a small effect include royal jelly,[25] fenugreek (small[26] or no effect[27]) and Tongkat Ali (promising effects, especially in older populations.[28] However, it remains unclear whether the fleeting bumps in testosterone caused by DNS boosters affect muscle mass.[29] It may have some therapeutic advantages for erectile dysfunction.[30] The available evidence suggests that testosterone-boosting supplements do not outperform 'testosterone-friendly'[31] foods such as garlic.[32]

Summary	Performance advantages	Health disadvantages/risks
	• Dietary protein above the recommended daily intake aids fat loss.[33] • Protein increases lean mass.[34] • Protein increases muscle protein synthesis.[35] • BCAAs attenuate fatigue and encourage recovery.[36] • Creatine augments lean mass and extends endurance.[37] • Most testosterone boosters have no clinical effect.[38]	• Low risk—Adverse effects of long-term over-consumption of protein include disorders of bone and calcium homeostasis; disorders of renal function; increased cancer risk; disorders of liver function; precipitated progression of coronary artery disease.[39] • Long-term high consumption of protein is low risk.[40]

Performance advantages	*Health disadvantages/risks*
Effects sought	Muscle mass Muscle preservation under caloric restriction Strength Power Recovery Fat loss
User profile	Bodybuilders Strength (and perhaps most) athletes Fat loss exercisers Older adults

CATEGORY 2. *Energy and endurance DNS*	Performance and energy enhancers Stimulants Aphrodisiacs Carbohydrates Electrolytes
Supplement	*Summary of effects*
Beta-alanine	Beta-alanine is a modified version of the amino acid alanine. It has been shown to enhance muscular endurance.[41] Supplementation can also improve moderate- to high-intensity cardiovascular exercise performance.
Caffeine	Caffeine is produced from coffee beans, but it can also be artificially synthesised. It has the same structure and effects irrespective of whether it is consumed via coffee, energy drinks, tea or pills. Caffeine constitutes the most used ergogenic aid in the world, and demonstrably works.[42] In short, caffeine allows more intense exercise for longer.[43] Caffeine is a powerful stimulant, and it can be used to improve physical strength and endurance. However, habitual use leads to a tolerance and a diminished effect, which can encourage higher dosages. Numerous studies demonstrate that caffeine enhances physiological responses to exercise, raises metabolic rate, increases heart rate, mobilises fat and delays fatigue.[44] The evidence suggests that caffeine is relatively safe— even health-promoting—as even low doses can be effective.[45] However, it can have an acute effect on children.[46]
Energy drinks	The main active constituents of energy drinks include varying amounts of caffeine, guarana extract, taurine and ginseng, although some add extra amino acids, vitamins and carbohydrates.[47] Energy drinks claim to improve performance by enhancing concentration and endurance while attenuating the fatigue and discomfort accompanying intense exercise or sleep deprivation. As a result, energy drinks enjoy tremendous popularity amongst users seeking sustained alertness or for better performance over repeated bouts of high effort. The largest market growth has been in the 18–25-year-old group, who commonly consume energy drinks as part of

Supplement	Summary of effects
	their late night social activities as well as in the early morning hours following heavy nights of socialising (and perhaps study).[48] Despite the proliferation of exotic ingredients found in energy drinks, the only verifiable effects come from caffeine, where excessive amounts can lead to toxicity.[49] In addition, most energy drinks contain high proportions of sugar (similar to soft drinks) and constitute a measurable contributor to obesity.[50] Of greater risk is the social prevalence of combining energy drinks with alcohol[51] (or in a pre-mixed version), cigarettes[52] and/or recreational drugs like ecstasy or amphetamines.[53]
HMB	HMB (short for β-hydroxy β-methylbutyrate) is a metabolite of the essential amino acid leucine, and purportedly helps prevent the breakdown of muscle protein, thereby delaying fatigue, promoting recovery and increasing power output. Although promising, early HMB studies revealed modest improvements in power output and muscular recovery in a few studies,[54] while other studies reported moderate[55] to no effects.[56] No serious risks to use have been observed.
Sodium bicarbonate	Sodium bicarbonate (household baking soda) increases serum levels of bicarbonate (produced by the kidneys) and 'buffers' acid production in the body. This acidosis is associated with physical fatigue during sustained exercise. As a result of diminishing acidosis, sodium bicarbonate leads to mild performance improvements, mostly due to a delay in the fatigue brought about through the accumulation of exercise-induced metabolic products in the body. Sodium bicarbonate has been shown to provide modest improvements to mid-distance sprints[57] and distance performances.[58] Some evidence has suggested that it leads to a boost in the muscular hypertrophy effects of resistance training.[59]
Nitrates (nitric oxide)	Nitrates and nitric oxide formulas claim to improve vasodilation and therefore assist blood flow to muscles. Cells release nitric oxide during exercise, releasing it into blood vessels and stimulating them to open wider to allow more blood to flow through.[60] As a result, nitric oxide substances are typically ingested prior to exercise with some effect, especially on endurance.[61]

Supplement	Summary of effects
	Studies have shown that the use of nitric oxide enhances exercise tolerance,[62] making moderate and heavy bouts a little easier[63] by improving muscular efficiency.[64] It also reduces blood pressure.[65] Some speculation has cautioned that nitric oxide could have deleterious effects on the kidney, but the most comprehensive and recent study concluded that is does not induce any specific kidney function modifications.[66] In terms of risk, it should be noted that many DNS products marketed as nitrates are designed as 'pre-workout' stimulants, and also contain high levels of caffeine. Many, in fact, contain a vast concoction of ingredients in addition to nitric oxide and caffeine, such as beta alanine, amino acids, antioxidants and carbohydrates.[67]
Aphrodisiacs	DNS sold as aphrodisiacs claim to stimulate sexual appetite or activity. For the most part, since the list of compounds associated with sexual enhancement is so long, studies remain largely unavailable. Nor can much be said for the theoretical mechanisms underpinning each substance's effects. Examples include horny goat weed, yohimbine and Tribulus terrestris. These substances have been empirically connected to mood changes, anxiety and hallucinations, as well as addictive behaviours[68] and psychotic symptoms.[69] However, establishing a clear causality to dosages and use is confounded by researchers' suspicions that the contents of each supplement varies considerably in concentration and may not even contain any of the substance at all. The role of the Internet appears to be extremely problematic for substance consistency:[70] for example, designer drugs have been found in supposedly herbal preparations.[71] The only available human studies have indicated that non-pharmaceutical aphrodisiacs do not work, or at best exhibit a marginal effect—a (probably) harmless waste of money. Mayo Clinic experts have warned that aphrodisiacs containing insect or plant extracts can be toxic.[72]
Carbohydrates	Carbohydrate supplements aim to replenish glycogen stores, build muscle and enhance the uptake

Supplement	Summary of effects
	of protein and amino acids.[73] Most comprise glucose, the preferred source of energy for muscles. Scores of studies since the early 1990s have measured the performance advantages of pre-loading, maintaining or replacing muscle glycogen with carbohydrate supplements. More recently, numerous meta-studies,[74] systematically reviewing hundreds of studies, have reported a confident performance benefit.[75] A clear conclusion is that the use of a range of carbohydrates (like glucose and fructose) is beneficial in prolonged exercise[76] and muscular hypertrophy,[77] although individual recommendations for athletes should be tailored according to each athlete's individual tolerance.[78] In addition, some studies have suggested that the supplements do not outperform normal foods like bananas[79] or fruit juice.[80] Like with most DNS, over-consumption can introduce gastric complaints[81] but otherwise should be considered low risk.
Electrolytes	Electrolyte replacements are supplements in the form of powders, tablets and pre-mixed drink products designed to deliver the targeted replacement of the electrolytes (such as sodium and potassium) lost through sweat. Typically, electrolyte supplements are used following intense exercise involving high levels of heat and perspiration. Under such conditions, electrolyte supplements help to restore fluid balance. According to a range of comprehensive studies, electrolyte supplements extend exercise capacity in the heat.[82] Since the loss of electrolytes is associated with dehydration, replacing essential fluids encourages faster recovery.[83] Most experts report little risk with moderate use, but note that electrolyte supplements are best used with more extreme physical performances.[84] However, electrolyte supplements are generally considered unnecessary[85] to maintain appropriate hydration during prolonged exercise in the heat.[86] For example, the use of additional replacement powders and pre-mixed drinks may not be necessary, as studies have shown that the combination of water and salt is sufficient to replenish the losses incurred through intense exercise during hot-weather endurance events.[87]

Summary	Performance advantages[88]	Health disadvantages[89]
	• Prolongs exercise • Increases alertness • Improves power • Accelerates recovery	• Generally low risk with moderate use • Over-stimulation risks with caffeine • Gastrointestinal complications with overuse
Effects sought	Longer athletic performance Better concentration despite fatigue Longer periods of wakefulness Faster recovery from exercise	
User profile	Athletes (serious and recreational): endurance and power Students Shift workers (especially security, military, medical)	

CATEGORY 3. *Fat and metabolism DNS*	Calorie-blockers Fat-burners
Supplement	*Summary of effects*
Calorie-blockers	Most DNS targeted at weight (fat) loss claim to: 1) increase energy expenditure (usually stimulants like caffeine); 2) modulate carbohydrate or fat metabolism; 3) increase satiety; or 4) block fat or carbohydrate absorption.[90] Calorie-blocker supplements work by preventing the intestinal uptake of either fatty acids or carbohydrates. They act on the pancreas to either avert the release of fat- and carbohydrate-digesting enzymes (such as lipase and amylase), or bind to the enzyme after release of the fat/carbohydrate itself, thereby stopping the enzyme from working.[91] Most of the DNS reviewed elicited no clinically meaningful effects in studies. This explains why calorie blockers are not particularly popular DNS, despite having been on the market in various forms since the early 1980s. Indeed, a history of calorie-blocking DNS reveals that they arise as fads only to rapidly fall out of circulation. For example, starch-blocker tablets do not inhibit the digestion and absorption of starch calories.[92] However, green coffee bean extract and white kidney bean extract may work to a limited extent for weight loss when employed in concert with dietary restrictions and/or exercise. When used alone, even the best weight loss DNS are largely ineffective.[93]
Green coffee beans	Green coffee bean extract supplements are made from the unroasted beans or raw seeds of coffee fruits. They contain high levels of chlorogenic acids, which reduce the absorption of fat and improve glucose metabolism and therefore blood sugar management.[94] Accounting for the caffeine content, green coffee bean extract has been linked to greater fat oxidation.[95] One meta-analysis of six recent studies reported that the effects of green coffee bean extract on body composition were modest but statistically significant, yet cautioned that each study contained limitations that precluded the supplement's endorsement.[96] At the same time, some studies have declared the long-term use of green coffee bean extract as effective because it accelerates glucose and fat metabolism.[97] Given the low risk nature of green coffee bean, the supplement extract appears to be a promising, if still unproven, DNS to mildly aid weight management.

Supplement	Summary of effects
Kidney bean extract	(White) kidney bean extract acts as a carbohydrate blocker that restricts the digestion of starches. By inhibiting starch digestion, undigested food remains in the gut and contributes fewer calories. However, because the starches are improperly absorbed, they can lead to gastrointestinal discomfort. Otherwise, kidney bean extracts are safe.[98] Like the other reviewed DNS in this category, kidney bean extract does work, albeit with a minor effect[99] that might not be worth the digestive trouble.[100]
Vinegar (apple cider vinegar)	Vinegar can help reduce hyperglycaemia, hyperinsulinaemia, hyperlipidaemia and obesity.[101] It works through several mechanisms, including the suppression of blood sugar, increase in fat oxidation and by supporting satiety.[102] Similarly, apple cider vinegar enjoys considerable anecdotal support as an insulin moderator, but few studies yet support its veracity.[103] One study suggested that vinegar worked as an appetite suppressant because it induced nausea.[104] Not only low-risk, apple cider vinegar is likely to be beneficial to general health.[105]
Fat burners	So-called fat-burning compounds aim to increase the rate of fat loss. Several actions are typically claimed, such as an increase in metabolic rate, a higher fat oxidation (more calories burned from fat compared to other sources) and an improved rate of fatty acid release.[106] According to the marketing delivered by the most recent fat-burning DNS, they can also work via 'uncoupling', where heat is raised inside fat cells, leading to their oxidation (no evidence supporting this effect could be located). The most effective fat burners do not operate directly upon fat cells. Rather, they create a hormonal effect (e.g. caffeine stimulates adrenaline) leading to a higher metabolic rate and therefore calorie expenditure.[107] It should be noted that these more effective fat burners are typically pharmaceutical-grade PIEDS (and are reviewed later). Several studies have recommended that fat-burners should be avoided because they are notoriously inconsistent in quality and may have differential effects on individuals. For example, fat-burners have been associated with liver[108] and adrenal damage,[109] although the risks of using 'real' pharmaceutical products (like ephedrine) far exceed those connected to herbal DNS compounds. The former are effective and risky, and the latter are ineffective and uncertain.[110]

Supplement	Summary of effects	
Conjugated linoleic acid (CLA)	It is believed that conjugated linoleic acid (CLA) enhances fat oxidation.[111] Very promising studies in animals,[112] suggesting that CLA was associated with rapid reductions in body fat, have led to a battery of human trials,[113] yet these studies have returned mixed effects on humans for fat loss.[114] At the same time, a few studies have shown some modest endurance performance benefits.[115] CLA supplementation is presently growing in popularity for weight loss, but the results are still discordant.[116] Small favourable effects have been recorded on appetite control.[117] Little is known about CLA's risk profile, but the early evidence so far points to negligible dangers.[118]	
Green tea	A substantive body of research supports the positive effects of green tea on general health and weight management. Most of the studies have focused on green tea's heavy concentration of epigallocatechin gallate (EGCG)—a potent polyphenol with antioxidant and anti-inflammatory properties—that also delivers a thermogenic and fat burning effect.[119] While highly positive from a health perspective, the studies on body composition have proven disappointing.[120] One recent comprehensive study reported that long-term green tea extract does not affect fat absorption and therefore body fat.[121] At present, the effects of green tea extract on fat loss appear to be modest at best.[122] Excessive use in a concentrated supplement form has been loosely linked with liver dysfunction.[123]	
Summary of Category 3 substances	*Performance advantages*	*Health disadvantages*
	• Marginal increases in fat burning, metabolism and caloric utilisation • Modest improvements in insulin and blood sugar management	• Gastrointestinal discomfort for some • Overuse might stress organs such as the liver and adrenals
Effects sought from Category 3 substances	Fat loss	
User profiles	Athletes seeking lower weight categories Bodybuilders, figure competitors, fitness models Image conscious gym users Adolescents seeking idealised bodies Middle-aged individuals seeking fat reduction	

DIETARY & NUTRITIONAL SUPPLEMENTS: Category 4

CATEGORY 4. *Immunity and inflammation DNS*	Antioxidants
	Immune boosters
	Joint health
	Vitamins and minerals
Overview	Oxidative stress has been connected to aging and chronic diseases.[124] A plethora of DNS claim antioxidant status, and their popularity has extended from those seeking general health and longevity benefits, to athletes and recreational trainers pursuing a recovery edge. Studies on antioxidant DNS have so far proven somewhat disappointing, as well as contradictory, failing to show any consistent improvements to health.[125] For example, while exercise-induced oxidative stress clearly improves insulin resistance and other positive adaptive responses, paradoxically, supplementation with antioxidants may preclude these health-promoting effects.[126] The experts are presently wondering whether antioxidant supplementation may undo some of the oxidative value of exercise. As a result, the conservative recommendation focuses instead on a diet rich in fruits and vegetables.[127]
	A recent study tested the effects of DNS antioxidants on sport performance. Beetroot juice worked, vitamin E, spiralina and quercetin returned marginal but favourable outcomes, and resveratrol (the active ingredient much touted in red wine) proved inconclusive.[128] Beneficial effects included small reductions in muscle fatigue and slightly better endurance. In another study, vitamin C turned out to be deleterious when used chronically, while blackcurrent juice showed mild promise in improving distance running times.[129] These studies have exposed a conundrum: antioxidants may hamper exercise adaptations, yet conversely they stimulate cell renewal and better vascular function.[130] Neither athletes nor the image-conscious are likely to find antioxidants decisively effective.
Supplement	*Summary of effects*
Curcumin	The antioxidant curcumin comes in the form of the yellow pigment contained in the curry spice, turmeric (and ginger in lesser amounts). It reportedly produces effects similar to other polyphenols, including an anti-inflammatory effect,[131] which might protect against some kinds of cancer,[132] as well as digestive benefits.[133] In terms of

Supplement	Summary of effects
	physical performance, curcumin seems to deliver positive, if small, results, with low risk. Numerous studies have shown that it will modestly fight muscle damage[134] and muscle soreness[135] from demanding exercise, especially when it involves heavy eccentric (lowering against resistance) contractions.[136] There is good reason to think that curcumin will work, but just not enough for visible results to display in the gym mirror.
Fish oil	Fish oil contains high levels of omega-3 fats (EPA and DHA), which presently enjoy an almost unrivalled popularity given the immense attention they have received as health-promoting substances. Supplements containing concentrated fish oil can help users maintain an optimum balance of omega-3 fats, leading to lower levels of systemic inflammation.[137] Some evidence shows that fish oils combat exercise-induced muscle damage[138] and aid in muscle recovery.[139] Other studies indicate that fish oil supplementation facilitates muscle protein synthesis.[140] In theory, fish oil should deliver nothing but benefits, but numerous studies have discovered that an alarmingly high proportion of fish oil DNS spoil prior to sale, relegating the source, quality, age and levels of refinement uncertain.[141]
Vitamin D	Vitamin D is a fat-soluble nutrient that has also enjoyed substantive positive publicity in recent times. Supplemental vitamin D has been linked to a suite of benefits including lengthier concentration, better immunity and reductions in the risks of cancer, heart disease and diabetes.[142] Athletes have become interested in vitamin D because testosterone levels increase following supplementation,[143] as does muscular recovery.[144] Meta-studies indicate that the health benefits of vitamin D are probably over-inflated, but most experts nevertheless encourage supplementation for those potentially deficient.[145]
Resveratrol	Resveratrol is a natural polyphenolic antioxidant that should, in theory, decrease LDL-cholesterol and prevent lipid oxidation.[146] On the one hand, DNS containing resveratrol have been linked to body fat reductions.[147] On the other hand, its effects were disappointing in trials of experienced athletes. For example, resveratrol should reduce the inflammatory response and delayed onset of muscle soreness after a marathon, but in fact did not help at all.[148] In another study, resveratrol supplementation actually blunted some of the good effects of exercise.[149]

Supplement	Summary of effects
	Also the compound helps improve glucose and insulin management in diabetics, but not in non-diabetics.[150] At best resveratrol might slightly reduce inflammation, but so far the results with active persons has been unimpressive.[151]
Glucosamine	Glucosamine DNS are claimed to improve joint function and lessen the pain and discomfort associated with heavy or long-term joint use. As a result, they have become a stalwart DNS for almost anyone from the recreational or serious athlete with complaining joints, to middle-aged and older individuals suffering from joint 'wear and tear'. Glucosamine is a component of the synovial fluid, tendons and ligaments in joints. Supplementation bolsters the natural quantities of synovial fluid and consequently aids joint function.[152]
	Glucosamine has been recommended in the treatment of joint pain for football players, but there is no evidence that its use can prevent joint injury or chronic pain.[153] However, it may slow cartilage degeneration.[154] Supplementation has been recommended for individuals with the cartilage degeneration that accompanies 'old knee injuries',[155] as well as for athletes with early osteoarthritis of the knee.[156] Although glucosamine will neither substantively improve performance nor make anyone look better, its low-risk positive effects will keep an individual on the sporting field or in the gym longer.
Vitamins and minerals	A review of all vitamins and minerals is impossible here, but many easily accessible online resources exist for potential users to consult.[157] The most 'potent' and popular individual vitamins and minerals have already been reviewed (e.g. vitamins C, D). However, it is worth noting that the majority of studies have reported no significant athletic benefits from vitamin and mineral DNS unless the user was deficient prior to consumption.[158] For this reason, sports physicians often prescribe certain vitamins and minerals to older athletes.[159] It is possible that combining certain minerals will provide a compounded effect, thereby delivering a minor effect on performance.[160] Although there might be little to lose other than the financial investment, the use of vitamin and mineral DNS augments general health but appear to have a negligible effect on performance or appearance.[161] Their general health roles are summarised below.[162]

Supplement	Summary of effects
	Vitamins
	A (Beta-Carotene) — Antioxidant used for skin, eyes, teeth, bones
	B Complex — Immune booster
	B1 (Thiamine) — Nervous system, growth and metabolism
	B2 (Riboflavin) — Formation of red blood cells and antibodies
	B3 (Niacin) — Skin and digestive system
	B5 (Pantothenic Acid) — Releases energy from fats and carbohydrates
	B6 (Pyridoxine) — Balances sodium and phosphorus
	B12 (Cyanocobalamin) — Metabolism and nervous system
	Biotin — Utilisation of other vitamins
	Choline — Nerves, liver and gall bladder function
	Folic Acid — Brain function and normal cell division
	Inositol — Hair growth
	PABA — Skin, hair and blood formation
	C (Ascorbic Acid) — Antioxidant for tissue repair
	D — Absorbs calcium and phosphorus
	E — Antioxidant
	K — For normal blood clotting
	Bioflavinoids — Capillaries and absorption of vitamin C
	Coenzyme Q10 — Immune system
	Minerals
	Calcium — Bones, teeth, nervous system and muscle
	Chromium — Insulin support for metabolism
	Copper — Formation of blood cells
	Iodine — Helps regulate metabolism
	Iron — Blood, immune system
	Magnesium — Utilisation of carbohydrates, fat and protein
	Manganese — Skeletal development and sex hormones
	Molybdenum — Iron transport from liver, cell function
	Potassium — Heart function, kidneys, nervous system
	Selenium — Promotes antibodies
	Zinc — Glands and immune system

DIETARY & NUTRITIONAL SUPPLEMENTS: Category 4 *continued*

Summary	Performance advantages	Health disadvantages
	• Extend endurance • Resist fatigue • Enhance recovery • Assist general health	• May reduce some of the benefits of exercise • Possible risk of contamination and quality variability
Effects sought	Decrease inflammation for recovery	
User profiles	Athletes at all levels Health users	

| CATEGORY 5. *Enhancement & augmentation* | Site injections

Skin pigmentation substances |
|---|---|
| *Overview* | The last decade has observed a radical increase in the use of human enhancement (HE) products for aesthetic purposes.[163] Of particular concern is the way the injection of HE products for muscle building, tanning and body 'site' enhancement has entered into mainstream fitness culture.[164] Although muscle fillers are not new, having been used for medical cosmetic purposes, the illegal and unsupervised use of muscle fillers has been rising alarmingly.[165] |
| *Supplement* | *Summary of effects* |
| Silicone | 'Silicone' remains a popular site enhancer, used by both women (typically for breast augmentation) and men (placed underneath muscle to bolster size). It is a relatively safe, inert liquid polymer characterised by thermal stability and durability. When administered by qualified cosmetic surgeons, silicone implants are considered quite safe. However, a considerable volume of use persists without medical oversight, often in unsterile locations such as homes, hotel rooms and pseudo-clinics, where untrained persons (so-called 'pumpers') inject users with a range of substances (e.g. loose silicone, cooking oil, tyre repair adhesive or industrial-strength silicone).[166] When delivered inexpertly, silicone- or oil-based substances can migrate from their injection site, sometimes leading to deformations or scarring.[167] At the most extreme, studies of silicone gone wrong have reported organ toxicity, as well as a range of associated and serious medical conditions with alarming names (including acute embolisation, chronic progressive granulomatous pneumonitis, acute alveolar haemorrhage and multiple small sub-acute brain white matter infarcts).[168] The subcutaneous injection of silicone in order to shape the face, breasts, hips and buttocks has been reported amongst women, transgendered and homosexual communities.[169] |
| Botox | The largest growth in site-enhancement injections includes the popular use of 'Botulinum toxin (BTXA)', commonly known as 'Botox'.[170] 'Botox' emerged from success in medical applications to treat migraine headaches and excessive sweating. The toxin works |

Supplement	Summary of effects
	by inhibiting the release of acetylcholine (ACH), temporarily reducing the tone—or hardness—of the muscles that have been injected. It therefore performs admirably as a transitory cosmetic remedy for facial wrinkles. Botox therapy is a safe and non-invasive substance that delivers an instant improvement in appearance.[171]
	Although a legitimate, legal and safe strategy for immediate appearance benefits when used by a licensed practitioner, the dark side of 'Botox' use once again concerns authenticity in both content and delivery. Versions of the substance—whether real or not—are easily accessible on the unregulated Internet and black market.[172] Evidence suggests that 'Botox' is regularly sourced without any guarantee as to its reliable content, and often administered by untrained individuals under conditions of questionable sterility and safety.[173] Numerous cases thread through the medical literature detailing serious infections caused by injections given by non-licensed practitioners.[174] Other documented side effects due to the improper use of 'Botox' (including contamination and improper application) include flu-like symptoms, visual disturbances, chronic fatigue, allergic reactions, pain, bruising and swelling.[175]
Synthol	Synthol is an injectable oil used by bodybuilders to make their muscles appear immediately bigger. The practice involves injecting the oil directly into a muscle belly to enlarge muscle volume, a practice known as 'fluffing'.[176] According to some research, bodybuilding users are drawn to Synthol for two reasons. First, they think that the practice does not involve the same risks as AAS, and second, they are attracted to its instantaneous results.[177]
	Synthol is widely available on the Internet. In fact, there is no medical option available for purchasing the substance, or for receiving administration by a trained health professional, so anyone seeking to employ the substance must locate the product and undertake the procedure him- or herself. The use of intramuscular injection of foreign substances for aesthetic purposes is well known.[178] A wide variety of studies report a cluster of health risks and side effects, including skin

Supplement	Summary of effects
	problems, nerve damage and oil-filled cysts at the injection site, as well as muscle damage and scar tissue development.[179] The effects of Synthol injection are immediately visible through the enlargement of the injection site. However, numerous case studies report a high chance of muscle deformity.[180] In some cases, an irreversible 'Swiss Cheese' appearance of the muscle can occur due to the development of. cysts that can leave the user with long-term muscle fibrosis.[181]
	Complications are usually localised to the site of injection, with medical reports specifying cases of irreversible muscle damage,[182] septic shock[183] and other lethal complications,[184] including death from asphyxia.[185]
Melanotan	Melanotan I and II initially became popular as a skin cancer-free tanning method that also sidestepped the cost and inconvenience of sunbeds or sunbathing. The drug imitates the naturally occurring hormones that stimulate melanin, leading to a darker skin tone.[186] Melanotan can be self-administered by injection or inhaled as a nasal spray.[187] Since its initial use, Melanotan has transformed into a so-called 'Barbie' drug due to the other side effects it creates as well as a tan, including weight loss and an elevated libido.[188] Studies have identified aesthetically driven females, body 'dysmorphics' and male bodybuilders as the principle user groups.[189]
	Little research has been undertaken concerning the long-term health implications of tan injections. Case reports describing growths, lesions and pigmentation abnormalities have been published.[190] In one study, an exotic dancer expressed positive experiences connected to her synthetic tanning, such as feelings of enhanced self-confidence and greater attractiveness emanating from her newly darkened skin.[191]
	According to research, a proliferation of cyber-forums exists prescribing everything associated with Melanotan use, including injection techniques, dosages, loading protocols, maintenance regimes and even tips for before and after photography.[192]

Summary	Performance advantages	Health disadvantages
	• None in general, but possible weight loss with Melanotan	• Skin problems • Cysts and lesions • Muscle damage and deformity • Septic shock • Scar tissue • Nerve damage
Effects sought	Enlarge muscle or shape body Darken skin	
User profiles	Bodybuilders Bodybuilders, figure competitors, fitness models Image-conscious gym users	

CATEGORY 6. *Anabolic agents PEDS*	Anabolic androgenic steroids (AAS: exogenous/ endogenous)
Substance	*Summary of effects*
Anabolic androgenic steroids (AAS)	Anabolic androgenic steroids (AAS) are versions of the male sex hormone, testosterone.[193] The term 'anabolic' refers to muscle-building properties, whilst 'androgenic' refers to male sexual characteristics. In a medical setting, AAS are used to treat conditions related to muscle wastage, or which undermine the body's natural hormone production. Testosterone and its popular metabolites, like dihydrotestosterone, instigate the changes associated with male development from adolescence to adulthood. Notably, these include increased muscle mass, facial and body hair, oily skin, acne and mood swings. AAS come in the form of 'exogenous' steroids, substances that cannot be produced by the body naturally, or 'endogenous' steroids, which can be produced by the body naturally. Testosterone has a substantive ergogenic effect that improves an athlete's performance through both enhanced recovery and greater muscle mass and strength.[194] It is also a substance of choice for the image-driven user. More recently a third category of anabolic agents, Selective Androgen Receptor Modulators (SARMs), have gained in popularity. Unlike testosterone, which has both anabolic and androgenic (masculinising) results,[195] SARMs maximise the former and minimise the latter, which means that there are fewer unwanted side effects. After entering the bloodstream, AAS help muscle cells to create and retain more protein through a process known as protein synthesis that, in turn, increases muscle size and strength. In addition, AAS can encourage muscle repair and growth by augmenting levels of free androgens, human growth hormone and insulin-like growth factor. Importantly, AAS also prevent muscles from entering a catabolic (breakdown) state as a result of extreme exercise, which allows users to train more frequently and more intensely without fear of

Substance	Summary of effects
Exogenous Anabolic androgenic steroids (AAS) Examples • Bolasterone • Boldenone • Danazol • Estosterone • Hydroxytestos- terone • Methandriol • Testosterone • Nandrolone • Oxabolone • Stanozolol • Stenbolone Endogenous Anabolic Androgenic Steroids (AAS) Examples • Androstenediol • Androstenedione • Dihydrotestos- terone • Prasterone • Testosterone Other Anabolic Agents: Examples • Clenbuterol • Selective Androgen Receptor Modulators (SARMs)	inadequate recovery. Since anabolic agents enhance protein synthesis enormously, they allow a large amount of muscle to be added in a short time. This means more size and strength, a reduction in recovery time after heavy exercise, and the ability to train harder and longer. SARMs have increased in popularity because they act directly on the so-called anabolic receptors that cause muscle growth. As a result, SARMs use leads to significantly fewer undesirable androgenic side effects that normally accompany a radical change to the hormone balance of the body.[196] For example, when males flood their bodies with extra testosterone, the natural response is an increase in the female hormone estrogen in order to compensate and reach a balance. SARMs therefore reduce the chances of stimulating female characteristics such as breast tissue development. (For females, the introduction of testosterone causes masculinising effects.) SARMs obviously remain of great interest to anyone interested in muscle development and recovery, with anti-doping detection tests presently under development.[197] Because AAS produce undesirable and dangerous side effects, their study cannot be undertaken in controlled clinical trials. Nevertheless, sufficient studies of user populations have yielded plenty of evidence about their dangers. In men, AAS have been shown to cause testicular atrophy, infertility and erectile dysfunction.[198] Once discontinued, users also commonly experience a loss of libido and episodes of major depression.[199] It is unclear whether AAS are addictive, but the limited data on lifetime usage rates (US data) are sufficiently alarming to indicate that either or both physiological and psychological addiction occurs.[200] Furthermore, an association has been documented between AAS use and affective and psychotic syndromes, as well as psychological dependence.[201]

Summary	Performance advantages[202]	Health disadvantages[203]
	• Muscular size and strength • Fat loss • Faster muscle recovery • Some endurance increase Medical uses • Anemia • Asthma • Bone pain from osteoporosis • Gonadal function decrease • Muscle loss • Postmenopausal symptoms • Puberty delay (males)	• Acne • Anger • Blood pressure elevation • Brain tissue damage • Cardiovascular disease risk • Depression and mood disturbances • Kidney tumours • Liver dysfunction • Serum cholesterol problems • Sudden death[204] • Tendon tearing Females • Abnormal menstrual cycles • Genital enlargement • Facial hair • Voice deepening Males • Breast enlargement • Impotence • Prostate enlargement • Sperm count decrease • Testicular atrophy • Some of the worst side effects can occur after AAS use has discontinued[205] • Risks appear to be higher for adolescents[206]
Effects sought	Muscle and strength gain Enhanced recovery Possible fat loss	
User profiles	Strength-based athletes Any athlete (including endurance) seeking faster recovery Bodybuilders Fitness and image-conscious users Young men	

PERFORMANCE ENHANCING DRUGS AND SUBSTANCES:
Category 7

CATEGORY 7. *Hormones PEDS*	Hormones and hormone-stimulating agents
Overview	Hormones are produced naturally in the body, effecting changes in organs and tissues, especially during growth periods and the transition from adolescence to adulthood. Although essential to development, hormones continue to be manufactured throughout adulthood. While their volume declines with age, various hormones support metabolism, muscle tissue growth/maintenance and the management (reduction) of adipose tissue during life. Human growth hormone (hGH), insulin and human chorionic gonadotrophin (HCG) are all commonly used for image and performance enhancing purposes. Since actual hormones can only be manufactured within a body, synthetic hormones have been produced to mimic the effects of those naturally occurring.[207] In addition to hormones, users may take hormone-stimulating agents. These work by either adding to the natural level of a hormone in the body, or by stimulating the production of naturally occurring hormones.[208] It should be noted that pharmaceutical-grade hormones are both extremely popular and expensive, which means that the market is flooded with cheap and dangerous counterfeits.
Substance	*Summary of effects*
Erythropoietin (EPO)	Erythropoietin, or EPO, is a glycoprotein hormone that regulates red blood cell production.[209] When taken as a performance enhancing substance, EPO substantially increases red blood cell numbers and, in so doing, the oxygen-carrying capacity of blood.[210] Naturally, the more oxygen in blood, the more that is delivered to muscles during aerobic activity. Because EPO boosts red blood cells, it has the potential to throw the 'haematocrit' (the ratio of blood cells to plasma) out of balance. In practice, the greater the number of red blood cells compared to plasma, the thicker blood becomes. For athletes seeking an endurance benefit from superior oxygen transport to muscles, more viscous blood from too much EPO can make the heart work harder in order to maintain circulation. EPO can therefore present a serious danger of blood clots, leading to strokes.

Summary	Performance advantages[211]	Health disadvantages[212]
	• Enhances fat oxidation • Enhances endurance • Improves cardiovascular and submaximal performance • Increases muscle mitochondria • Increases muscle myoglobin concentration • Improves muscle recovery • Improves memory *It is possible that the performance enhancing effects of EPO are exaggerated.[213] <u>Medical uses</u> • Anaemia from kidney failure • HIV • Some cancers	• Potential death • Deep vein thrombosis • Heart attack • Myocardial infarction • Pulmonary embolism • Stroke • Thrombosis
Human growth hormone — somatotropin (STH)	Human growth hormone is a naturally occurring peptide hormone produced in the pituitary gland, and is responsible for stimulating growth, cell reproduction and regeneration.[214] Somatrophin (rhGH) describes pharmaceutical human growth hormone synthesised with the use of recombinant DNA technology; it is biologically equivalent to hGH of pituitary origin. For athletes, the results can include increases in muscle growth and strength, and greater production of red blood cells to improve the blood's ability to carry oxygen.[215] Growth hormone operates in a synergistic way with testosterone, leading to increased muscle size and strength while simultaneously diminishing fat. It may also reduce sensitivity to insulin and raise blood sugar levels.[216] Growth hormone is probably the most anabolic hormone known.[217] Claims of growth hormone's benefits include increases in muscle mass and strength, especially in conjunction with AAS, and accelerated tissue healing and recovery from injury or hard training.[218] Studies in healthy young adults have also demonstrated a performance benefit with GH and IGF-1.[219]	

Substance	Summary of effects	
	No studies have conclusively demonstrated that growth hormone alone improves performance, although there is some evidence connecting exercise with growth hormone levels.[220] Although not definitively correlated to actual performance, hGH has been shown to decrease body fat.[221] Indeed, the studies in which GH was shown to have the greatest positive effect on athletic performance were in anabolic steroid users.[222] A systematic review of 27 studies comprising a total of 303 healthy adults, in whom the effects of GH on various measures of athletic performance were analysed (such as muscle strength and endurance), concluded that claims that hGH enhances physical performance are not supported by the scientific literature.[223] In the largest study of nearly 100 recreational athletes, neither muscle strength nor muscle power were affected by eight weeks of blinded GH administration.[224]	
Summary	*Performance advantages*	*Health disadvantages*[225]
	• Muscle growth • Muscle repair • Body fat reduction • Strength increases • Protein synthesis increase Medical uses • Cosmetic anti-ageing • Growth hormone deficiencies • Turner's syndrome	• Unwanted tissue growth (acromegaly) • Arthritis • Brain swelling • Cardiomyopathy • Congestive heart failure • Coronary artery disease • Cruetzfeldt–Jakob disease • Diabetes mellitus • Hypoglycaemia • Hypothyroidism • Impotence • Osteoporosis
Gonadotrophins Examples • Luteinizing Hormone (LH) • Human chorionic gonadotrophin (hCG)	Human chorionic gonadotrophin (hCG) is a glycoprotein hormone produced in large amounts during pregnancy. Male athletes can use pharmaceutical preparations of hCG to stimulate testosterone production.[226] It also reduces or prevents the testicular atrophy and natural testosterone shut-down that accompanies lengthy and high-dosage courses of AAS.[227] Excessive use of hCG may lead to gynaecomastia[228] (male breast tissue enlargement) and may hinder the	

Substance	Summary of effects	
	return to normal testicular function in males.[229] Other side effects may include headaches, restlessness, fatigue and mood changes,[230] and hypogonadism (when the body's sex glands produce little or no sex hormones).[231] Luteinizing hormone (LH) is produced in the anterior pituitary gland. It regulates the testes in men and the ovaries in women. Luteinising hormone controls sex steroid production (testosterone in men and oestradiol in women), and is therefore used as a performance enhancing substance for the same purposes as hCG. In some cases, hCG and LT can mask the presence of AAS.	
Summary	Performance advantages	Health disadvantages
	• Increases testosterone • Prevents testicular damage • Masking agent for AAS Medical uses • Female infertility	• Similar effects as AAS
Insulin Insulin-like growth factors (e.g. IGF-1) Mechano growth factors (MGFs)	Insulin is a powerful peptide hormone that promotes glucose utilisation and protein synthesis through the regulation of sugar metabolism. When taken in conjunction with testosterone, it is widely considered by athletes—and especially strength athletes and bodybuilders—to be the most anabolic hormone available. Too much insulin at one time can lead to hypoglycaemic shock, coma and even death. Insulin stimulates protein anabolism, glucose uptake and glycogen storage in muscle.[232] In short, it increases muscle anabolism and improves the amount of glucose available to muscles during exercise. The hormone is both anabolic and anti-catabolic (stops muscle breakdown) to skeletal muscle tissue, which explains its popularity in elite sport and bodybuilding. Hypoglycaemia, which occurs when blood glucose levels fall dangerously low, can be a side effect of insulin use. In a study of bodybuilders using insulin,	

Substance	Summary of effects	
	57% reported symptoms consistent with hypoglycaemia.[233] Users remain at a high risk for going into a state of severe hypoglycaemia during sleep, during which, of course, carbohydrates cannot be consumed to offset the impact. The result can be a coma or worse.[234] Other studies have concluded that insulin abuse can indeed cause unconsciousness, coma and death.[235] Insulin-like growth factors, or IGFs, are also peptide hormones secreted by the liver. Athletes and image users employ IGF-1 for its anabolic effect on muscle. Mechano Growth Factors (MGFs) are related substances, derived from IGF-1. Like IGF-1, MGFs assist in tissue repair after damage, making them favourable substances for muscular recovery following heavy exercise. IGF-I promotes cell proliferation and supports some of the metabolic pathways that play a role in carcinogenesis. IGF-I abuse can increase cancer risk.[236]	
Summary	*Performance advantages*	*Health disadvantages*
	• Decreases body fat (with AAS) • Muscle growth (with AAS) • Reduces protein breakdown Medical uses • Diabetes	• Risk of death • Brain damage • Coma • Hypoglycaemia • Nausea • Shortness of breath • Increases cancer risk
Corticotrophins Example • Adrenocortico-tropic hormone (ACTH)	Corticotrophins, or adrenocorticotropic hormone (ACTH), stimulate the adrenal gland to secrete corticosterone, which in turn moderate the stress hormone system, including cortisol. Corticotrophin also acts on other areas within the brain and can suppress appetite, increase anxiety and improve memory and focus.[237] These effects manipulate the body's response to stressful experiences. Athletes can take advantage by stimulating their bodies to perform at higher levels, especially during competition. ACTH has been shown to diminish fatigue during submaximal physical efforts.[238]	

Summary of Category 7 substances	Performance advantages	Health disadvantages
	• Heightens focus • Increases adrenal corticosteroid levels • Aids injury recovery Medical uses • Spasm control in children	• Psychological over-stimulation • Connective tissue softening • Stomach irritation and ulcers • Weakening of muscles
Effects sought from Category 7 substances	Increase muscle size, strength and endurance Reduce body fat Increase body's tolerance to stress	
User profiles	Serious strength, power and endurance athletes Serious bodybuilders, powerlifters and fitness athletes/models	

PERFORMANCE ENHANCING DRUGS AND SUBSTANCES:
Category 8

CATEGORY 8. Hormonal manipulators PEDS	Hormone antagonists & modulators
Overview	Hormone antagonists and modulators, or anti-estrogenic substances, act by either decreasing the amount of the female hormone oestrogen in the body or by blocking the oestrogen receptors. Testosterone's effects on muscle mass and strength are proportional to dose.[239] Hormone manipulators increase testosterone indirectly—that is, not by introducing more exogenous testosterone but by either stimulating its production or reducing other hormones that restrict its production, like oestrogen.[240] Aromatase inhibitors, Selective Oestrogen Receptor Modulators (SERMs), oestrogen blockers and myostatin blockers are all used by athletes and image enhancers seeking to 1) increase testosterone without actually taking it directly, and 2) help correct the 'paradoxical' feminisation side effects of using AAS. Hormone antagonists and modulators may increase the risks of cancer, but their long-term effects remain unknown.[241]
Substance	*Summary of effects*
Aromatase inhibitors Examples • Aminoglutethi-mide • Anastrozole • Exemestane • Formestane • Letrozole • Testolactone	Oestrogen blockers significantly increase testosterone levels in men, leading to the same advantages that accompany the use of exogenous testosterone.[242] Elite athletes almost exclusively use this class of hormone manipulators as a means to bypass tests for banned androgens that directly raise testosterone.[243] Individuals pursuing an image effect—and who do not need to pass anti-doping tests—will simply choose the more direct path of using AAS or growth hormones. No research has been undertaken investigating the risks of aromatase inhibitor abuse. In clinical settings, aromatase inhibitors have been linked to side effects including asthenia (lethargy), headache, nausea, peripheral oedema (swelling), fatigue, vomiting and dyspepsia (digestion problems).[244]

Substance	Summary of effects	
Selective oestrogen receptor modulators (SERMs) Examples • Raloxifene • Tamoxifen • Toremifene Other anti-estrogenic substances Examples • Clomiphene • Cyclofenil • Fulvestrant	Tamoxifen citrate is a non-steroidal anti-oestrogenic drug, or a SERM.[245] It functions as an oestrogen in some tissues while blocking its action in others.[246] In male bodybuilders and athletes, tamoxifen citrate and SERMs in general are commonly used to counter the side effects caused by elevated oestrogen levels accompanying the use of certain AAS. SERMs can also increase blood testosterone levels in men.[247] Both male and female athletes and image enhancers employ anti-oestrogens like Tamoxifen and Clomiphene. Males use Tamoxifen in concert with AAS to reduce the likelihood of breast tissue growth. By reducing oestrogen, the drug also increases the effects of testosterone.[248] Female strength athletes can use Tamoxifen to block oestrogen receptors, increasing levels of both natural and artificial testosterone.	
Myostatin inhibitors (Growth differentiation factor 8—GDF-8) Example • Follistatin	Myostatin (growth differentiation factor 8, GDF-8) is a protein connected to a gene that has a strong influence on an individual's propensity for muscular development.[249] A key role of myostatin is to withhold muscle growth from continuing beyond natural needs.[250] Therefore, blocking myostatin leads to greater muscle mass and strength, although it can also have the side effect of making muscles more vulnerable to injury.[251] As a relatively new class of drugs, few human studies are available to reveal its effects. However, studies do show that animals lacking myostatin, and livestock given substances like Follistatin that block myostatin, have significantly larger muscles.[252]	
Summary	Performance advantages	Health disadvantages
	• Anabolic effects • Strength increases • Reduction of AAS side effects Medical uses • Breast cancer • Infertility (females) • Muscular dystrophy (myostatin inhibitors)	• Abdominal cramps • Increases in cancer risk • Libido swings • Speech difficulties

Effects sought	Offset side effects of excess testosterone from AAS use
	Increase strength and muscle mass
User profiles	Bodybuilders and strength athletes

PERFORMANCE ENHANCING DRUGS AND SUBSTANCES:
Category 9

CATEGORY 9. *Beta-2 agonists* PEDS	Beta-2 agonists
Substance	*Effects*
<u>Examples</u> • Clenbuterol • Formoterol • Salbutamol • Salbutarnol • Salmeterol • Terbutaline	Beta-2 agonists are prescribed to treat asthma because they dilate the bronchial passages by relaxing the muscles constraining the airway. However, they also have a stimulant effect. Furthermore, when injected, Beta-2 Agonists stimulate anabolic effects, generating greater muscle mass while diminishing body fat at the same time.[253] Given their widespread availability, easy prescription, moderate cost and low chance of contamination or inauthenticity, clenbuterol in particular has become a substance of choice for image-conscious users. Clenbuterol hydrochloride is an anti-asthma medication, but can be used to treat a range of conditions such as asthma, hypertension, cardiovascular shock, arrhythmias, migraine headaches and anaphylactic shock. However, clenbuterol produces a substantial shift in lean body mass, increasing muscle at the same time as diminishing fat.[254] As a result, the drug represents a popular 'holy grail' substance for image-motivated users. The possible side effects of clenbuterol hydrochloride use include shaky hands, insomnia, sweating, increased blood pressure and nausea. Overdose may be accompanied by rapid breathing, blood pressure irregularities, irregular heartbeat, unconsciousness, trembling, shaking, panic and extreme restlessness, plus severe nausea, vomiting or diarrhoea.[255] At its most severe, clenbuterol hydrochloride has the potential for fatal overdose.[256] Beta-2 agonists are more commonly inhaled as bronchodilators in the treatment of asthma. While some studies report that bronchodilators do not necessarily deliver advantages in endurance performance for non-asthmatics,[257] it is nevertheless plausible that their respiratory effects might bolster performance in other, less well-understood, ways. After all, asthmatic athletes outperform their non-asthmatic peers at the Summer and Winter Olympics.[258] For example, compared to inhaled

Substance	Summary of effects	
	beta-2 agonists, the oral administration of calbutarnol enhances muscle strength and endurance.[259] Risks of overuse and abuse revolve around cardio-pulmonary toxicity.[260]	
Summary	*Performance advantages*	*Health disadvantages*
	• Increases in aerobic performance • Reduces body fat • Increases in muscle mass Medical uses • Asthma • Chronic obstructive pulmonary disease	• Anxiety • Dizziness • Headache • Insomnia • Cramps • Nausea • Palpitations • Psychological over-stimulation
Effects sought	Increase in muscle mass while decreasing body fat Improvement in bronchodilation	
User profiles	Bodybuilders and fitness athletes	

CATEGORY 10. *Masking agents* PEDS	Diuretics and masking agents
Overview	Masking agents are substances that can be used to conceal the presence of a prohibited (under the WADA conventions governing elite sport) substance in urine or other samples. As a result, they can fall into a range of drug categories depending upon their intended medical usages. For example, aromatase inhibitors and selective oestrogen receptor modulators (SERMs) are sometimes taken to mask the gynaecomastia caused by anabolic steroid abuse.[261] Diuretics provide another example, as they are used to dilute urine samples. They can also help athletes remove weight prior to weight-controlled events like wrestling, boxing, weightlifting, horse racing and martial arts.[262]
Substance	*Summary of effects*
Epitestosterone	One common substance used as a masking agent is epitestosterone. Epitestosterone (E) is an inactive form of testosterone that may serve as a storage substance, or as a precursor to testosterone that is converted to active testosterone.[263] In males, a natural ratio exists between the hormones testosterone and epitestosterone.[264] When an athlete takes exogenous testosterone, his or her testosterone level increases but the epitestosterone level does not, throwing out the usual ratio. Drug tests measure for discrepancies in the ratio. Athletes can re-balance the ratio by taking additional epitestosterone.[265] The technique appears to be used by both male and female athletes.[266] It does not improve performance.
Diuretics Examples • Acetazolamide • Chlorthalidone • Etacrynic acid • Metolazone • Spironolactone • Triamterene	Diuretics increase urine flow and sodium excretion, which have the effect of changing the body's fluid composition. As a result, athletes use diuretics to eliminate water for rapid weight loss and to conceal the presence of other banned substances.[267] In addition, fitness, bodybuilding and figure competitors regularly employ diuretics during their pre-competition dehydration process in order to better reveal their physiques on stage, or for photo shoots. Misuse can

Substance	Summary of effects	
Other substances Examples • Epitestosterone • Probenecid • Alpha-reductase inhibitors • Plasma expanders	lead to dangerous levels of dehydration and abnormal concentrations of electrolytes like potassium, chloride, calcium, bicarbonate or magnesium.[268]	
Summary	*Performance advantages*	*Health disadvantages*
	• Hides banned substances • Dilutes banned substances in samples • Weight loss Medical uses • Heart failure • High blood pressure	• Blood pressure problems • Cramps • Dehydration • Electrolyte imbalances • Headaches • Heart failure • Kidney failure • Muscle cramps • Nausea
Effects sought	Cover the use of other banned substances Dilute urine Accelerate weight (water) loss	
User profiles	Elite athletes Bodybuilding and fitness competitors and models Athletes seeking to reduce weight for a performance category	

CATEGORY 11A. *Stimulants PEDS*	Stimulants
Overview	Stimulants encompass numerous substances affecting an increase in concentration, alertness and physical performance through greater central nervous system activation. Anyone interested in gaining a physical or mental advantage can use stimulants to improve attention, escalate psychological readiness, fight fatigue and pain, suppress appetite and amplify aggressiveness.[269] The greatest danger of stimulant use comes from their hyper-stimulation of the nervous system, which can cause a range of systemic problems from mild heart palpitations and sweating to heart attack and stroke.[270]
	Examples of common stimulants span from ephedrine (and its derivatives) and amphetamines, to adrenaline and cocaine, although only the former pair are regularly employed for performance or image purposes. Athletes use stimulants to augment their physical arousal, while the image-conscious use them to lose fat.
Substance	*Summary of effects*
Ephedrine (and pseudo-ephedrine)	Ephedrine is a stimulant drug that enhances the release of norepinephrine, resulting in a reaction similar to the body's natural release of adrenaline. Ephedrine can produce side effects such as shaky hands, headaches, tremors, sweating, rapid heartbeat, dizziness and anxiety. Users focused on image effects find ephedrine appealing because it dampens appetite and increases caloric expenditure. In fact, ephedrine is often included in prescription appetite suppressants.
	The long-term abuse of ephedrine has been linked to myocardial damage and ventricular arrhythmia[271] (abnormal rapid heart rhythms), as well as hypertension accompanying the severe increases in heart rate, blood pressure and cardiac output that come with use.[272] Not only is ephedrine highly risky, it is reportedly used in concert with other stimulants like caffeine, which elevates the danger further.[273] One concern according to one major meta-study is that ephedrine is on the top 10 list of most popular substances to use in concert with AAS.[274]

Substance	Summary of effects
	Pseudo-ephedrine is a stimulant that can be purchased over the counter to relieve symptoms of nasal and sinus congestion. It has a similar composition to ephedrine and other amphetamines, and therefore delivers comparable ergogenic effects.[275] Although the use of pseudo-ephedrine is considered sufficiently safe for non-prescription access, its effects are dose dependent and there is plenty of evidence that performance and image users exceed recommended dosages.
Amphetamines	Amphetamine is a central nervous system 'psychostimulant' used in the treatment of attention deficit hyperactivity disorder, narcolepsy and obesity.[276] It is popular because it can enhance alertness and aggression, but also offsets both physical and mental fatigue. Common adverse effects include restlessness, headache, insomnia, anxiety and the potential for psychological instability.[277]
	Athletes employ amphetamines due to their ability to increase exercise duration by masking fatigue.[278] Image users favour amphetamines because they increase plasma free fatty acid (FFA) concentrations,[279] which spares skeletal muscle glycogen, delays fatigue and mobilises fat. Increased concentrations of plasma FFA may have a skeletal muscle glycogen-sparing effect and thereby delay the onset of fatigue.[280]
	Amphetamines remain popular for recreational use, not just because they can prolong a party but because they replace fatigue with euphoria and augmented senses.[281] There is no medical justification for the use of amphetamines in sport.[282]
CATEGORY 11B. *Cognitive enhancers PEDS*	Cognitive enhancers
Substance	Summary of effects
Methylphenidate	Methylphenidate is a stimulant related to amphetamine[283] and acts as a catecholamine reuptake inhibitor.[284] It increases concentrations of dopamine and noradrenaline by blocking their reuptake.[285] This drug is generally used

Substance	Summary of effects
	in the treatment of attention deficit hyperactivity disorder (ADHD). For cognitive enhancement in healthy individuals, it is said to be the drug of choice for students.[286]
	There is some evidence to suggest that methylphenidate can increase working memory, memory consolidation and information processing in healthy individuals, but research has produced mixed results.[287] As a result, it is difficult to draw a firm conclusion on its effects.[288]
	In general, stimulants consumed in large doses can cause seizures, psychosis and cardiovascular events.[289] Potential side effects of methylphenidate include headaches, hypertension, anxiety, depression and anaphylactic reactions.[290] The use of this drug by healthy individuals is also of concern due to the potential for dependence and abuse.[291]
Modafinil	Modafinil is a 'wakefulness promoting agent' used in the treatment of sleepiness during the day associated with narcolepsy, sleep apnoea and shift worker disorder.[292] The precise manner in which modafinil works is not completely known.[293] However, it has been suggested that it may have effects similar to methylphenidate on the reuptake of dopamine and norephinephrine. In addition, it may have an augmenting effect on neurotransmitters such as serotonin and glutamate.[294]
	In sleep-deprived individuals, even a single dose of modafinil has been shown to enhance executive function, but for individuals who are not sleep deprived, the effect of modafinil is somewhat ambiguous.[295] It has also been suggested that the effect of this drug is somewhat dependent on the baseline IQ of individuals.
	Potential adverse reactions include headaches, dizziness, gastrointestinal complaints, tachycardia and palpitations, nervousness and restlessness. For non-sleep-deprived individuals, insomnia may also be a side effect.[296]
Racetams	Racetams are derivatives of the parent compound piracetam, and share a common pyrrolidone structure. Variations include aniracetam and oxiracetam. Along with piracetam, they have produced results that suggest

Substance	Summary of effects	
	nootropic benefits in impaired patients through positive modulation of glutamate receptors in neurons.[297] Piracetam, aniracetam and oxiracetam have been used in the treatment of impaired cognitive function, including dementia.[298,299] Aniracetam has been shown in studies to be relatively well tolerated by patients with mild to moderate senile dementia,[300] while oxiracetam has had similar tolerance results with Alzheimer's.[301]	
Other examples • Adrenaline • Cocaine • Ephedrine • Mesocarb • Methamphetamine (D-) • Oxilofrine • Sibutramine • Strychnine • Tsuaminoheptane	*Performance advantages* • Increases aggression • Increases alertness and attention • Reduces fatigue • Reduces pain • Lowers weight Medical uses • Allergies • Asthma • Attention deficit hyperactivity disorder • Headache • Nasal congestion	*Health disadvantages* • Addiction/withdrawal • Aggressiveness • Anxiety • Blood pressure fluctuations • Cardiac arrhythmia • Convulsions • Dehydration • Heart attack • Insomnia • Stroke
Effects sought	Promotes concentration and alertness Reduces fatigue and enhances energy Fat loss	
User profiles	Competitive athletes (endurance and aggression-oriented sports) Adolescents seeking weight loss Fitness competitors and models Recreational party goers Students	

CATEGORY 12. *Pain and pleasure narcotics PEDS*	Narcotics/analgesics
Overview	Narcotic analgesics act on the brain and spinal cord to reduce or remove pain, and often come with 'feel good' side effects both mild and significant. The potential benefits to athletes from narcotics include euphoria and an increased pain threshold.[302] Athletes can use analgesics to reduce the pain from injury or just to endure more uncomfortable training and its consequences.[303] They allow users to function longer during discomfort and get back to training or performance faster by supressing pain from injury. However, narcotic analgesics only conceal the pain brought about by overuse or injury, and do nothing to affect the underlying causes. As a result, it is easy for users to unknowingly increase the severity of their injuries because the normal pain feedback has been masked. Codeine, morphine and pethidine are common examples. Typically cited adverse effects include a false sense of security or even invulnerability, perceptions of physical ability exceeding reality, an inability to recognise injury and physical or psychological dependence.[304] According to studies, younger athletes in high-contact sports (e.g. wrestling and football) are at a higher risk of the non-medical use of prescription opioids (NUPOs).[305] NUPOs in young athletes constitute a serious concern given that prescription opioid misuse has been revealed as a strong risk factor for heroin use.[306] The non-medical use of narcotics and analgesics by adolescents in competitive sport and recreational settings is growing because these are feel-better, feel-good drugs.[307]
Substance	*Summary of effects*
Morphine Codeine Vicodin	Morphine is a powerful analgesic that increases tolerance to pain, thereby improving physical performance.[308] A less powerful but more common analgesic, codeine, is present in many commonly used headache, pain relief, cough and cold preparations.[309] Its use is ubiquitous at all levels of physical activity, from professional sport[310] to amateur recreation.[311]

PERFORMANCE ENHANCING DRUGS AND SUBSTANCES:
Category 12 *continued*

Substance	Summary of effects
	Another common opioid painkiller is Vicodin, which has been associated with non-medical use in sport and heavy physical exercise.[312]
Cortisone (corticosteroid) injections	Corticosteroids are synthetic drugs that closely resemble cortisol, a hormone that is naturally produced in the adrenal glands. Corticosteroid medicines include cortisone, prednisone and methylprednisolone, which are used medically to treat certain rheumatologic diseases. Corticosteroids are different from the male hormone-related steroid compounds used for building muscle and strength, but nevertheless appear to be common in serious sport in order to relieve pain and inflammation, often in targeted areas through injections.[313] Injections are common treatments for knee osteoarthritis[314] and other joint problems such as 'golfer's' and 'tennis' elbow.[315] For example, one study revealed that in patients with adhesive capsulitis (painful, stiff shoulder), a single corticosteroid injection offered faster pain relief and earlier improvement of shoulder function and motion compared with oral non-steroidal anti-inflammatory drugs (NSAIDs).[316]

Administering local anaesthetics or corticosteroid injections to professional athletes in order to get them back on the field faster remains controversial. However, the medical literature recommends corticosteroid injections as a safe and effective therapeutic intervention for treating muscle strains and ligament sprains in order to enable athletes to return to competition earlier.[317] The caveat on this endorsement is oversight and administration by a qualified medical practitioner, who will not be swayed by pressure to return an athlete to competition through injection when it might undermine his or her longer-term joint health. Some serious allergic reactions to corticosteroids have been documented, but these seem to be rare.[318] Repeated doses of corticosteroids can weaken joints.[319] |
| Cough mixtures, antihistamines | Many cough suppressants contain Dextromethorphan (DMX), a safe substance when used at prescribed dosages, but also a powerful and risky hallucinogenic when used for recreational purposes. |

Substance	Summary of effects
	It may also be addictive[320] and is easy to acquire, especially online.[321] A mixture of codeine cough syrup with alcohol and/or a soft drink known as 'purple drank' has gained media attention in recent years as a drug associated with professional athletes.[322] In high dosages, cough syrups containing DMX can induce euphoria, altered time perception, feelings of floating, visual disturbance, tactile, visual and auditory hallucination, disorientation and increased perceptual awareness. However, these sometimes pleasant and relaxing symptoms belie its darker effects, ranging from gastrointestinal discomfort to brain toxicity.[323]

Other examples	Performance advantages	Health disadvantages
• Buprenorphine • Diamorphine (heroin) • Methadone • Morphine • Pethidine • Sleeping pills • Vicodin	• Reduces pain • Increases in pain threshold • Sensation of euphoria and well-being Medical uses • Treatment of pain	• Addiction/withdrawal • Balance and coordination loss • Cardiovascular distress • Concentration problems • Injury risk increase • Nausea and vomiting

Alcohol		
Alcohol	Alcohol is a central nervous system depressant that acts by reducing the speed of the brain and body. Its uses in sport can include the reduction of anxiety and physical tremors. Alcohol can also improve relaxation. However, alcohol's intoxicating effects are well known to diminish judgement while increasing inappropriate feelings of psychological well-being, self-confidence and aggression. Acute alcohol consumption impairs muscle hypertrophy and recovery.[324]	

Example	Performance advantages	Health disadvantages
• Ethanol	• Reduces anxiety • Sedative Medical uses • Antiseptic	• Addiction/withdrawal • Cirrhosis of the liver • Judgement impairment • Memory loss • Poor muscular coordination impairment

PERFORMANCE ENHANCING DRUGS AND SUBSTANCES:
Category 12   *continued*

Effects sought	Pain and inflammation suppression
	Faster return after injury
	Feel-good high
User profiles	Professional athletes
	Recreational pleasure seekers

CATEGORY 13. Adrenal manipulators PEDS	Beta-blockers
Overview	Beta-blockers inhibit the effects of adrenaline (epinephrine), a hormone produced by the adrenal glands that stimulates the central nervous system. In blocking adrenaline, beta-blockers decrease blood pressure, heart rate, muscle tremors and anxiety.[325] Since beta-blockers relax the body and its musculature, they offer advantages to athletes seeking to steady their hands or concentrate on fine-motor activities. These effects may be performance enhancing in sports where increased steadiness is desirable, such as archery, shooting, snooker, darts and golf.[326] Conversely, however, beta-blockers undermine the body's capacity to perform strenuous activities, as the heart cannot meet the needs of muscles and other internal systems. As a result, they have a deleterious effect on most physical performance—including strength, power and endurance—because they inhibit the body's ability to respond to exercise load and intensity.[327] Beta-blockers appear to be of little use to those individuals prioritising image, although they can be employed by anyone for recreational purposes such as relaxation.
Substance	*Summary of effects*
<u>Examples</u> • Acebutolol • Betaxolol • Celiprolol • Esmolol • Metipranolol • Oxprenolol • Propranolol • Sotalol • Timolol	Studies indicate that beta-blockers do deliver improved performances in physical activities demanding steady, slow and concentrated movements. For example, in one seminal study the beta-blocker Metoprolol was tested against a placebo on 33 marksmen, leading to a 13.4% improvement in performance.[328] Sports psychiatrists have reported some concern that beta-blockers such as Propranolol can be used for relaxation, outside any form of sporting performance.[329] While the image-conscious have little to gain by using beta-blockers to augment their physiques, there remains the potential for the substances to be employed for recreational reasons. Some research has demonstrated that the administration of beta-blockers can in fact have an adverse effect on mood, including the worsening of depressive states.[330] A comprehensive meta-study

Substance	Summary of effects	
	covering 55 studies investigating the cognitive side effects of beta-blockers reported contradictory outcomes, with the exception that the drugs seem to universally increase sedation.[331] It is possible that beta-blockers may increase a user's predisposition to exertion-caused hyperthermia, which means that it becomes easier to dangerously overheat.[332]	
Summary	*Performance advantages*	*Health disadvantages*
	• Muscle relaxant • Reduces tremors Medical uses • Sedatives for anxiety • Heart problems • High blood pressure • Migraine	• Severe blood pressure reduction • Severe heart rate decrease • Physical performance decrease • Insomnia • Fatigue
Effects sought	Steady hands and reduce tremors Relaxation	
User profiles	Controlled-skill sport players Recreational relaxation-seekers	

PERFORMANCE ENHANCING DRUGS AND SUBSTANCES:
Category 14

CATEGORY 14. *Psychoactives* *PEDS*	Cannabinoids	
Substance	*Summary of effects*	
Example • Marijuana	Cannabinoids are a class of 'psychoactive' substances refined from the cannabis plant that affect cognition, including feelings of relaxation. As a calmative, cannabinoids can be used to recover from heavy exertion.[333] However, as substances with psychoactive properties, cannabinoids can lead to psychological disturbances and are dangerously addictive.[334] Studies have demonstrated that the use of cannabinoids can reduce anxiety, but they do not have ergogenic potential in sports activities. For example, the psychoactive stimulant tetrahydrocannabinol (THC) can decrease cardiac and psychomotor output, leading to lowered athletic performance.[335] Only 15 published studies have investigated the effects of THC in association with exercise protocols. Of these studies, none showed any improvement in aerobic performance.[336] On the other hand, the literature concerning the recreational use of cannabinoids is prodigious (but is not reviewed here). Other than their possible use for relaxation and recreation, cannabinoids have no attraction to individuals interested in looking better.	
Summary	*Performance advantages*	*Health disadvantages*
	• Muscle relaxant • May assist recovery • Medical uses • Calmative	• Addiction/withdrawal • Anxiety and panic • Concentration problems • Psychological disturbances • Motor skill difficulties
Effects sought	Relaxation and calming, 'feeling good' Possible use for high performance-induced stress	
User profiles	Elite athletes seeking stress reduction Recreational pleasure-seekers	

PERFORMANCE ENHANCING DRUGS AND SUBSTANCES:
Category 15

CATEGORY 15. *Anti-inflammatories* *PEDS*	Glucocorticosteroids	
Substance	*Summary of effects*	
Examples • Acetonide Dexamethasone • Fluticasone • Hydrocortisone • Prednisolone • Triamcinolone	Glucocorticosteroids are anti-inflammatory steroid hormones produced in the adrenal glands. In a medical context, glucocorticosteroids are used to treat the pain and inflammation accompanying asthma, hay fever, tissue inflammation and rheumatoid arthritis.[337] In addition to the anti-inflammatory and painkilling effects, athletes can use glucocorticosteroids to induce a feeling of well-being despite injury or illness.[338] The use of glucocorticosteroids bolsters exercise performance by reducing muscle fatigue during intense, sustained exercise.[339] Their anti-inflammatory and analgesic effects might also inhibit sensations of muscle pain during effort, further elevating the fatigue threshold.[340] The side effects of acute and short-term glucocorticosteroids use are less severe than those reported with chronic treatment.[341] In fact, sustained use can cause impaired insulin sensitivity, hyperglycaemia, lymphopenia, hyperarousal and altered energy store metabolism.[342] More generally, studies have suggested that long-term use or abuse of glucocorticosteroids can incur a wide range of organ problems including musculoskeletal, gastrointestinal, cardiovascular, endocrine, neuropsychiatric, dermatologic, ocular and immunologic side effects.[343] Corticosteroids act as potent anti-inflammatory drugs and have been used in various sport settings for the treatment of both acute and chronic injuries. If clinically justified with medical oversight, however, corticosteroid treatment for sports injuries is considered relatively low risk.[344]	
Summary	*Performance advantages*	*Health disadvantages*
	• Reduce inflammation • Reduce pain • Induce feelings of well-being	• Fluid retention • Hyperglycaemia • Mood changes • Risk of injury increases

PERFORMANCE ENHANCING DRUGS AND SUBSTANCES:
Category 15 *continued*

Summary	Performance advantages	Health disadvantages
	Medical uses • Arthritis • Asthma • Inflammation • Allergies	
Effects sought	Reduction in pain and inflammation Accelerate return from injury	
User profiles	Elite and serious athletes	

Conclusion

On the surface, physical performance involves several broad requirements including skill, power, strength, endurance and recovery.[345] Correspondingly, the major ergogenic PIEDS classes deliver effects aligned to one or more of these elements. For example, all physical activities requiring a skills base benefit from PIEDS that curtail anxiety and tremors, improve concentration and attention and offset distraction and mental fatigue. Activities dependent upon the performance of explosive, anaerobic power benefit mostly from PIEDS stimulating muscle mass and strength. Those activities favouring sustained aerobic endurance benefit from PIEDS that resist fatigue and promote cardiovascular effort, including blood oxygenation. Finally, physical activities demanding constant or repeated performances benefit from the tissue-regenerating effects of hormones, as well as the pain-controlling advantages of analgesics. In addition, individuals with appearance-oriented physical objectives utilise PIEDS that match their collective body image ideals. These predominantly revolve around increasing muscle mass (and sometimes strength to impress), and decreasing fat. However, to optimise appearance, users commonly augment their regimes with PIEDS that accelerate recovery, repair injury, combat pain, improve joint function, stimulate energy, darken skin, decrease inflammation, extend effort, amplify metabolism, induce relaxation and even hide PIEDS usage. And, if all of these PIEDS fail to work— or if they are not enough to satisfy a user's body image goals—a person can always simulate real tissue with physical, sometimes surgical, augmentations.

Notes

1   Luiking, Y. C., Deutz, N. E., Memelink, R. G., Verlaan, S. & Wolfe, R. R. (2014). Postprandial muscle protein synthesis is higher after a high whey protein, leucine-enriched supplement than after a dairy-like product in healthy older people: A randomized controlled trial. *Nutrition Journal*, *13*(1), 9–23.

2 Pasiakos, S. M., McLellan, T. M. & Lieberman, H. R. (2015). The effects of protein supplements on muscle mass, strength, and aerobic and anaerobic power in healthy adults: a systematic review. *Sports Medicine, 45*(1), 111–131.

3 Verreijen, A. M., Verlaan, S., Engberink, M. F., Swinkels, S., de Vogel-van den Bosch, J. & Weijs, P. J. (2015). A high whey protein-, leucine-, and vitamin D-enriched supplement preserves muscle mass during intentional weight loss in obese older adults: a double-blind randomized controlled trial. *The American Journal of Clinical Nutrition, 101*(2), 279–286.

4 Pasiakos, S. M., Lieberman, H. R. & McLellan, T. M. (2014). Effects of protein supplements on muscle damage, soreness and recovery of muscle function and physical performance: a systematic review. *Sports Medicine, 44*(5), 655–670; Wolfe, R. R. (2000). Protein supplements and exercise. *The American Journal of Clinical Nutrition, 72*(2), 551s–557s.

5 Joy, J. M., Lowery, R. P., Wilson, J. M., Purpura, M., De Souza, E. O., Wilson, S. M., Kalman, D. S., Dudeck, J. E. & Jäger, R. (2013). The effects of 8 weeks of whey or rice protein supplementation on body composition and exercise performance. *Nutrition Journal, 12*(1), 86–93.

6 Snijders, T., Smeets, J. S., van Vliet, S., van Kranenburg, J., Maase, K., Kies, A. K., Verdijk, L. B. & van Loon, L. J. (2015). Protein ingestion before sleep increases muscle mass and strength gains during prolonged resistance-type exercise training in healthy young men. *The Journal of Nutrition, 145*(6), 1178–1184.

7 Pasiakos, S. M., Lieberman, H. R. & McLellan, T. M. (2014). Effects of protein supplements on muscle damage, soreness and recovery of muscle function and physical performance: A systematic review. *Sports Medicine, 44*(5), 655–670.

8 Andersen, L. L., Tufekovic, G., Zebis, M. K., Crameri, R. M., Verlaan, G., Kjær, M., Suetta, C., Magnusson, P. & Aagaard, P. (2005). The effect of resistance training combined with timed ingestion of protein on muscle fiber size and muscle strength. *Metabolism, 54*(2), 151–156; Kerksick, C. M., Rasmussen, C. J., Lancaster, S. L., Magu, B., Smith, P., Melton, C., Greenwood, M., Almada, A. L., Earnest, C. P. & Kreider, R. B. (2006). The effects of protein and amino acid supplementation on performance and training adaptations during ten weeks of resistance training. *The Journal of Strength & Conditioning Research, 20*(3), 643–653.

9 Pedersen, A. N., Kondrup, J. & Børsheim, E. (2013). Health effects of protein intake in healthy adults: A systematic literature review. *Food & Nutrition Research, 57*(1), 1–29.

10 Graf, S., Egert, S. & Heer, M. (2011). Effects of whey protein supplements on metabolism: Evidence from human intervention studies. *Current Opinion in Clinical Nutrition & Metabolic Care, 14*(6), 569–580.

11 Aristoy, M. C. & Toldrá, F. (2012). Essential amino acids. In M. C. Aristoy & F. Toldrá (eds), *Handbook of Analysis of Active Compounds in Functional Foods* (pp. 3–25). Boca Raton, FL: CRC Press.

12 Williams, M. (2005). Dietary supplements and sports performance: Amino acids. *Journal of the International Society of Sports Nutrition, 2*(2), 63–67.

13 Wu, G. (2009). Amino acids: Metabolism, functions, and nutrition. *Amino Acids, 37*(1), 1–17.

14 Børsheim, E., Tipton, K. D., Wolf, S. E. & Wolfe, R. R. (2002). Essential amino acids and muscle protein recovery from resistance exercise. *American Journal of Physiology–Endocrinology and Metabolism, 283*(4), E648–E657.

15 Kerksick, C. M., Rasmussen, C. J., Lancaster, S. L., Magu, B., Smith, P., Melton, C., Greenwood, M., Almada, A. L., Earnest, C. P. & Kreider, R. B. (2006). The effects of protein and amino acid supplementation on performance and training adaptations during ten weeks of resistance training. *The Journal of Strength & Conditioning Research, 20*(3), 643–653; Willoughby, D. S., Stout, J. R. & Wilborn, C. D. (2007). Effects of resistance training and protein plus amino acid supplementation on muscle anabolism, mass, and strength. *Amino Acids, 32*(4), 467–477.

16 Jafari, H., Ross, J. B. & Emhoff, C. A. W. (2016). Effects of branched-chain amino acid supplementation on exercise performance and recovery in highly endurance-trained athletes. *The FASEB Journal, 30*(1), lb683–lb683; Waldron, M., Whelan, K., Jeffries, O., Burt, D., Howe, L. & Patterson, S. D. (2017). The effects of acute branched-chain amino acid supplementation on recovery from a single bout of hypertrophy exercise in resistance-trained athletes. *Applied Physiology, Nutrition, and Metabolism*, 10.1139/apnm–2016-0569.

17 Tipton, K. D. & Wolfe, R. R. (2004). Protein and amino acids for athletes. *Journal of Sports Sciences, 22*(1), 65–79.

18 Candow, D. G., Chilibeck, P. D., Burke, D. G., Mueller, K. D. & Lewis, J. D. (2011). Effect of different frequencies of creatine supplementation on muscle size and strength in young adults. *The Journal of Strength & Conditioning Research, 25*(7), 1831–1838; Hoffman, J., Ratamess, N., Kang, J., Mangine, G., Faigenbaum, A. & Stout, J. (2006). Effect of creatine and β-alanine supplementation on performance and endocrine responses in strength/power athletes. *International Journal of Sport Nutrition and Exercise Metabolism, 16*(4), 430–446.

19 Benavidez, G. A., Detomasi, N. & Hart, P. D. (2016). Short-term effects of creatine supplementation on physical fitness measures in moderately active college-aged females: A randomized placebo-controlled pilot study. *Journal of Physical Activity Research, 1*(1), 15–19; Theodorou, A. S., Paradisis, G. & Smpokos, E. (2017). The effect of carbohydrate augmented creatine supplementation on anaerobic performance. *Biology and Sport, 34*(2), 169–175.

20 Riesberg, L. A., Weed, S. A., McDonald, T. L., Eckerson, J. M., & Drescher, K. M. (2016). Beyond muscles: The untapped potential of creatine. *International Immuno-pharmacology, 37*, 31–42.

21 Dorrell, H., Gee, T. & Middleton, G. (2016). An update on effects of creatine supplementation on performance: a review. *Sports Nutrition and Therapy, 1*(1), e107–e107; Deldicque, L. & Francaux, M. (2016). Potential harmful effects of dietary supplements in sports medicine. *Current Opinion in Clinical Nutrition & Metabolic Care, 19*(6), 439–445; Herriman, M., Fletcher, L., Tchaconas, A., Adesman, A. & Milanaik, R. (2017). Dietary supplements and young teens: Misinformation and access provided by retailers. *Pediatrics*, e20161257.

22 Bell, A., Dorsch, K. D., Mccreary, D. R. & Hovey, R. (2004). A look at nutritional supplement use in adolescents. *Journal of Adolescent Health, 34*(6), 508–516.

23 Raja, R. R. (2016). Nutraceuticals and cosmeceuticals for human beings–An overview. *American Journal of Food Science and Health, 2*(2), 7–17.

24 Hassan, A. A. (2009). Effect of royal jelly on sexual efficiency in adult male rats. *Iraqi Journal of Veterinary Sciences, 23*(2), 155–160.

25 Yang, A., Zhou, M., Zhang, L., Xie, G., Chen, H., Liu, Z. & Ma, W. (2012). Influence of royal jelly on the reproductive function of puberty male rats. *Food and Chemical Toxicology, 50*(6), 1834–1840.

26 Sinha, R., Rauniar, G. P., Panday, D. R. & Adhikari, S. (2015). Fenugreek: pharmacological actions. *World Journal of Pharmacy and Pharmaceutical Sciences, 5*(1), 1481–1489; Wankhede, S., Mohan, V. & Thakurdesai, P. (2016). Beneficial effects of fenugreek glycoside supplementation in male subjects during resistance training: A randomized controlled pilot study. *Journal of Sport and Health Science, 5*(2), 176–182.

27 Bushey, B., Taylor, L. W., Wilborn, C. W., Poole, C., Foster, C. A., Campbell, B., Kreider, R. & Willoughby, D. S. (2009). Fenugreek extract supplementation has no effect on the hormonal profile of resistance-trained males. *International Journal of Exercise Science: Conference Proceedings, 2*(1), 13.

28 Henkel, R. R., Wang, R., Bassett, S. H., Chen, T., Liu, N., Zhu, Y. & Tambi, M. I. (2014). Tongkat Ali as a potential herbal supplement for physically active male and female seniors—A pilot study. *Phytotherapy Research, 28*(4), 544–550.

29 Talbott, S. M., Talbott, J. A., George, A. & Pugh, M. (2013). Effect of Tongkat Ali on stress hormones and psychological mood state in moderately stressed subjects. *Journal of the International Society of Sports Nutrition*, *10*(1), 28–33.

30 Kotirum, S., Ismail, S. B. & Chaiyakunapruk, N. (2015). Efficacy of Tongkat Ali (*Eurycoma longifolia*) on erectile function improvement: Systematic review and meta-analysis of randomized controlled trials. *Complementary ThernPEDS in Medicine*, *23*(5), 693–698.

31 Incledon, T. (2016). Top 6 Testosterone Friendly Foods. *Month, 2016.*

32 Nishimatsu, H., Kitamura, T., Yamada, D., Nomiya, A., Niimi, A., Suzuki, M., Fujimura, T., Fukuhara, H., Nakagawa, T., Enomoto, Y. & Kume, H. (2014). Improvement of symptoms of aging in males by a preparation LEOPIN ROYAL containing aged garlic extract and other five of natural medicines–comparison with traditional herbal medicines (Kampo). *The Aging Male*, *17*(2), 112–116.

33 Baer, D. J., Stote, K. S., Paul, D. R., Harris, G. K., Rumpler, W. V. & Clevidence, B. A. (2011). Whey protein but not soy protein supplementation alters body weight and composition in free-living overweight and obese adults. *The Journal of Nutrition*, *141*(8), 1489–1499; Graf, S., Egert, S. & Heer, M. (2011). Effects of whey protein supplements on metabolism: Evidence from human intervention studies. *Current Opinion in Clinical Nutrition & Metabolic Care*, *14*(6), 569–580; Hoffman, J. R., Ratamess, N. A., Tranchina, C. P., Rashti, S. L., Kang, J., & Faigenbaum, A. D. (2009). Effect of protein-supplement timing on strength, power, and body-composition changes in resistance-trained men. *International Journal of Sport Nutrition and Exercise Metabolism*, *19*(2), 172–185; Pal, S., Ellis, V. & Dhaliwal, S. (2010). Effects of whey protein isolate on body composition, lipids, insulin and glucose in overweight and obese individuals. *British Journal of Nutrition*, *104*(5), 716–723.

34 Andersen, L. L., Tufekovic, G., Zebis, M. K., Crameri, R. M., Verlaan, G., Kjær, M., Suetta, C., Magnusson, P. & Aagaard, P. (2005). The effect of resistance training combined with timed ingestion of protein on muscle fiber size and muscle strength. *Metabolism*, *54*(2), 151–156; Kerksick, C. M., Rasmussen, C. J., Lancaster, S. L., Magu, B., Smith, P., Melton, C., Greenwood, M., Almada, A. L., Earnest, C. P. & Kreider, R. B. (2006). The effects of protein and amino acid supplementation on performance and training adaptations during ten weeks of resistance training. *The Journal of Strength & Conditioning Research*, *20*(3), 643–653.

35 Reitelseder, S., Agergaard, J., Doessing, S., Helmark, I. C., Lund, P., Kristensen, N. B., Frystyk, J., Flyvbjerg, A., Schjerling, P., van Hall, G. & Kjaer, M. (2011). Whey and casein labeled with L-[1-13C] leucine and muscle protein synthesis: effect of resistance exercise and protein ingestion. *American Journal of Physiology-Endocrinology and Metabolism*, *300*(1), E231–E242; Tipton, K. D., Elliott, T. A., Cree, M. G., Wolf, S. E., Sanford, A. P. & Wolfe, R. R. (2004). Ingestion of casein and whey proteins result in muscle anabolism after resistance exercise. *Medicine and Science in Sports and Exercise*, *36*, 2073–2081.

36 Blomstrand, E. (2006). A role for branched-chain amino acids in reducing central fatigue. *The Journal of Nutrition*, *136*(2), 544S–547S.

37 Chwalbińska-Moneta, J. (2003). Effect of creatine supplementation on aerobic performance and anaerobic capacity in elite rowers in the course of endurance training. *International Journal of Sport Nutrition and Exercise Metabolism*, *13*(2), 173–183.

38 Bell, A., Dorsch, K. D., Mccreary, D. R. & Hovey, R. (2004). A look at nutritional supplement use in adolescents. *Journal of Adolescent Health*, *34*(6), 508–516.

39 Delimaris, I. (2013). Adverse effects associated with protein intake above the recommended dietary allowance for adults. *ISRN Nutrition.*

40 Song, M., Fung, T. T., Hu, F. B., Willett, W. C., Longo, V. D., Chan, A. T. & Giovannucci, E. L. (2016). Association of animal and plant protein intake with all-cause and cause-specific mortality. *JAMA Internal Medicine*, *176*(10), 1453–1463.

41 Glenn, J. M., Gray, M., Stewart Jr, R. W., Moyen, N. E., Kavouras, S. A., DiBrezzo, R., Turner, R., Baum, J. I. & Stone, M. S. (2016). Effects of 28-day beta-alanine

supplementation on isokinetic exercise performance and body composition in female masters athletes. *The Journal of Strength & Conditioning Research*, *30*(1), 200–207; Jagim, A. R., Wright, G. A., Brice, A. G. & Doberstein, S. T. (2013). Effects of beta-alanine supplementation on sprint endurance. *The Journal of Strength & Conditioning Research*, *27*(2), 526–532: Quesnele, J. J., Laframboise, M. A., Wong, J. J., Kim, P. & Wells, G. D. (2014). The effects of beta-alanine supplementation on performance: A systematic review of the literature. *International Journal of Sport Nutrition and Exercise Metabolism*, *24*(1), 14–27.

42 Momaya, A., Fawal, M. & Estes, R. (2015). Performance-enhancing substances in sports: A review of the literature. *Sports Medicine*, *45*(4), 517–531.

43 Cruz, R. S. D. O., de Aguiar, R. A., Turnes, T., Guglielmo, L. G. A., Beneke, R. & Caputo, F. (2015). Caffeine affects time to exhaustion and substrate oxidation during cycling at maximal lactate steady state. *Nutrients*, *7*(7), 5254–5264.

44 Pasman, W. J., Van Baak, M. A., Jeukendrup, A. E. & De Haan, A. (1995). The effect of different dosages of caffeine on endurance performance time. *International Journal of Sports Medicine*, *16*(4), 225–230; Tallis, J., Duncan, M. J. & James, R. S. (2015). What can isolated skeletal muscle experiments tell us about the effects of caffeine on exercise performance? *British Journal of Pharmacology*, *172*(15), 3703–3713.

45 Spriet, L. L. (2014). Exercise and sport performance with low doses of caffeine. *Sports Medicine*, *44*(2), 175–184.

46 Turley, K. R. (2016). Effects of caffeine on exercise responses and performance in children and youth. *American Journal of Lifestyle Medicine*, *10*(6), 417–421.

47 Higgins, J. P., Tuttle, T. D. & Higgins, C. L. (2010, November). Energy beverages: content and safety. *Mayo Clinic Proceedings*, *85*(11), 1033–1041. London: Elsevier.

48 Gunja, N. & Brown, J. A. (2012). Energy drinks: Health risks and toxicity. *Medical Journal of Australia*, *196*(1), 46–49.

49 Reissig, C. J., Strain, E. C. & Griffiths, R. R. (2009). Caffeinated energy drinks— A growing problem. *Drug and Alcohol Dependence*, *99*(1), 1–10.

50 Riddell, L. & Keast, R. (2007). Is caffeine in soft drinks really necessary? *Medical Journal of Australia*, *187*(11–12), 655–655.

51 Verster, J. C., Aufricht, C. & Alford, C. (2012). Energy drinks mixed with alcohol: Misconceptions, myths, and facts. *International Journal of General Medicine*, *5*, 187–198.

52 Weldy, D. L. (2010). Risks of alcoholic energy drinks for youth. *The Journal of the American Board of Family Medicine*, *23*(4), 555–558.

53 Miller, K. E. (2008). Energy drinks, race, and problem behaviors among college students. *Journal of Adolescent Health*, *43*(5), 490–497.

54 Durkalec-Michalski, K. & Jeszka, J. (2015). The efficacy of a β-hydroxy-β-methyl-butyrate supplementation on physical capacity, body composition and biochemical markers in elite rowers: A randomised, double-blind, placebo-controlled crossover study. *Journal of the International Society of Sports Nutrition*, *12*(1), 31–42.

55 Wilson, J. M., Lowery, R. P., Joy, J. M., Andersen, J. C., Wilson, S. M., Stout, J. R., Duncan, N., Fuller, J. C., Baier, S. M., Naimo, M. A. & Rathmacher, J. (2014). The effects of 12 weeks of beta-hydroxy-beta-methylbutyrate free acid supplementation on muscle mass, strength, and power in resistance-trained individuals: a randomized, double-blind, placebo-controlled study. *European Journal of Applied Physiology*, *114*(6), 1217–1227.

56 Wilson, J. M., Fitschen, P. J., Campbell, B., Wilson, G. J., Zanchi, N., Taylor, L., Wilborn, C., Kalman, D. S., Stout, J. R., Hoffman, J. R. & Ziegenfuss, T. N. (2013). International society of sports nutrition position stand: beta-hydroxy-beta-methylbutyrate (HMB). *Journal of the International Society of Sports Nutrition*, *10*(1), 6–20.

57 Brisola, G. M. P., Miyagi, W. E., da Silva, H. S. & Zagatto, A. M. (2015). Sodium bicarbonate supplementation improved MAOD but is not correlated with 200- and 400-m running performances: A double-blind, crossover, and placebo-controlled study. *Applied Physiology, Nutrition, and Metabolism*, *40*(9), 931–937.

58 Hobson, R. M., Harris, R. C., Martin, D., Smith, P., Macklin, B., Elliott-Sale, K. J. & Sale, C. (2014). Effect of sodium bicarbonate supplementation on 2000-m rowing performance. *International Journal of Sports Physiology and Performance*, *9*(1), 139–144.

59 Carr, B. M., Webster, M. J., Boyd, J. C., Hudson, G. M. & Scheett, T. P. (2013). Sodium bicarbonate supplementation improves hypertrophy-type resistance exercise performance. *European Journal of Applied Physiology*, *113*(3), 743–752.

60 Besco, R., Sureda, A., Tur, J. A., & Pons, A. (2012). The effect of nitric-oxide-related supplements on human performance. *Sports Medicine*, *42*(2), 99–117.

61 Lansley, K. E., Winyard, P. G., Bailey, S. J., Vanhatalo, A., Wilkerson, D. P., Blackwell, J. R., . . . & Jones, A. M. (2011). Acute dietary nitrate supplementation improves cycling time trial performance. *Medicine and Science in Sports and Exercise*, *43*(6), 1125–1131.

62 Jones, A. M. (2014). Dietary nitrate supplementation and exercise performance. *Sports Medicine*, *44*(1), 35–45.

63 Pawlak-Chaouch, M., Boissière, J., Gamelin, F. X., Cuvelier, G., Berthoin, S. & Aucouturier, J. (2016). Effect of dietary nitrate supplementation on metabolic rate during rest and exercise in human: A systematic review and a meta-analysis. *Nitric Oxide*, *53*, 65–76.

64 Wylie, L. J., Mohr, M., Krustrup, P., Jackman, S. R., Ermidis, G., Kelly, J., . . . & Jones, A. M. (2013). Dietary nitrate supplementation improves team sport-specific intense intermittent exercise performance. *European Journal of Applied Physiology*, *113*(7), 1673–1684.

65 Siervo, M., Lara, J., Ogbonmwan, I. & Mathers, J. C. (2013). Inorganic nitrate and beetroot juice supplementation reduces blood pressure in adults: A systematic review and meta-analysis. *The Journal of Nutrition*, *143*(6), 818–826.

66 Carpentier, A., Stragier, S., Bréjeon, C. & Poortmans, J. R. (2015). Nitrate supplementation, exercise, and kidney function: Are there detrimental effects? *Medicine and Science in Sports and Exercise*, *47*(7), 1519–1522.

67 Bloomer, R. J., Farney, T. M., Trepanowski, J. F., McCarthy, C. G., Canale, R. E. & Schilling, B. K. (2010). Comparison of pre-workout nitric oxide stimulating dietary supplements on skeletal muscle oxygen saturation, blood nitrate/nitrite, lipid peroxidation, and upper body exercise performance in resistance trained men. *Journal of the International Society of Sports Nutrition*, *7*(1), 16–31.

68 Corazza, O., Martinotti, G., Santacroce, R., Chillemi, E., Di Giannantonio, M., Schifano, F. & Cellek, S. (2014). Sexual enhancement products for sale online: Raising awareness of the psychoactive effects of yohimbine, maca, horny goat weed, and Ginkgo biloba. *BioMed Research International*, dx.doi.org/10.1155/2014/841798.

69 Wong, M. K., Darvishzadeh, A., Maler, N. A. & Bota, R. G. (2016). Five supplements and multiple psychotic symptoms: A case report. *The Primary Care Companion for CNS Disorders*, *18*(1), 10.4088/PCC.15br01856.

70 Israel, J. & Laborde, E. L. (2016). Alternative and internet drugs that affect sexual function. In *Contemporary Treatment of Erectile Dysfunction* (pp. 137–148). London: Springer International.

71 Venhuis, B. J., Blok-Tip, L. & De Kaste, D. (2008). Designer drugs in herbal aphrodisiacs. *Forensic Science International*, *177*(2), e25–e27.

72 Bauer, B. A. (2017). Do natural aphrodisiacs actually work? Retrieved from www. mayoclinic.org/healthy-lifestyle/sexual-health/expert-answers/natural-aphrodisiacs/faq-20058252

73 Tarnopolsky, M. A., Bosman, M., Macdonald, J. R., Vandeputte, D., Martin, J., & Roy, B. D. (1997). Postexercise protein-carbohydrate and carbohydrate supplements increase muscle glycogen in men and women. *Journal of Applied Physiology*, *83*(6), 1877–1883.

74 Devries, M. C. & Phillips, S. M. (2014). Creatine supplementation during resistance training in older adults-a meta-analysis. *Medicine and Science in Sports and Exercise*, *46*(6), 1194–1203.

Vandenbogaerde, T. J. & Hopkins, W. G. (2011). Effects of acute carbohydrate supplementation on endurance performance. *Sports Medicine, 41*(9), 773–792.

75 Stellingwerff, T. & Cox, G. R. (2014). Systematic review: Carbohydrate supplementation on exercise performance or capacity of varying durations. *Applied Physiology, Nutrition, and Metabolism, 39*(9), 998–1011.

76 Gomes, R. V., Moreira, A., Coutts, A. J., Capitani, C. D. & Aoki, M. S. (2014). Effectof carbohydrate supplementation on the physiological and perceptual responses to prolonged tennis match play. *The Journal of Strength & Conditioning Research, 28*(3), 735–741.

77 Tarpenning, K. M., Wiswell, R. A., Hawkins, S. A. & Marcell, T. J. (2001). Influence of weight training exercise and modification of hormonal response on skeletal muscle growth. *Journal of Science and Medicine in Sport, 4*(4), 431–446.

78 Jeukendrup, A. (2014). A step towards personalized sports nutrition: Carbohydrate intake during exercise. *Sports Medicine, 44*(1), 25–33.

79 Nieman, D. C., Gillitt, N. D., Henson, D. A., Sha, W., Shanely, R. A., Knab, A. M., Cialdella-Kam, L. & Jin, F., 2012. Bananas as an energy source during exercise: A metabolomics approach. *PLoS One, 7*(5), e37479.

80 Prasertsri, P., Roengrit, T., Kanpetta, Y., Tong-un, T., Muchimapura, S., Wattanathorn, J. & Leelayuwat, N. (2013). Cashew apple juice supplementation enhanced fat utilization during high-intensity exercise in trained and untrained men. *Journal of the International Society of Sports Nutrition, 10*(1), 13–19.

81 Peters, H. P., Van Schelven, F. W., Verstappen, P. A., De Boer, R. W., Bol, E. D., Erich, W. B., Van Der Togt, C. R. & De Vries, W. R. (1993). Gastrointestinal problems as a function of carbohydrate supplements and mode of exercise. *Medicine and Science in Sports and Exercise, 25*(11), 1211–1224.

82 James, L. J., Mears, S. A. & Shirreffs, S. M. (2015). Electrolyte supplementation during severe energy restriction increases exercise capacity in the heat. *European Journal of Applied Physiology, 115*(12), 2621–2629.

83 Khong, T. K., Selvanayagam, V. S., Sidhu, S. K. & Yusof, A. (2017). Role of carbohydrate in central fatigue: a systematic review. *Scandinavian Journal of Medicine & Science in Sports, 27*(4), 376–384.

84 Ranchordas, M. K., Hudson, S. & Thompson, S. W. (2017). Nutrition for extreme sports. In F. Feletti (ed.), *Extreme Sports Medicine* (pp. 15–28). London: Springer International.

85 Potgieter, S. (2013). Sport nutrition: A review of the latest guidelines for exercise and sport nutrition from the American College of Sport Nutrition, the International Olympic Committee and the International Society for Sports Nutrition. *South African Journal of Clinical Nutrition, 26*(1), 6–16.

86 Hoffman, M. D. & Stuempfle, K. J. (2016). Is sodium supplementation necessary to avoid dehydration during prolonged exercise in the heat? *The Journal of Strength & Conditioning Research, 30*(3), 615–620.

87 Del Coso, J., González-Millán, C., Salinero, J. J., Abián-Vicén, J., Areces, F., Lledo, M., Lara, B., Gallo-Salazar, C. & Ruiz-Vicente, D., 2016. Effects of oral salt supplementation on physical performance during a half-ironman: A randomized controlled trial. *Scandinavian Journal of Medicine & Science in Sports, 26*(2), 156–164.

88 Tokish, J. M., Kocher, M. S. & Hawkins, R. J. (2004). Ergogenic aids: a review of basic science, performance, side effects, and status in sports. *The American Journal of Sports Medicine, 32*(6), 1543–1553.

89 Finnegan, D. (2003). The health effects of stimulant drinks. *Nutrition Bulletin, 28*(2), 147–155.

90 Torres-Fuentes, C., Schellekens, H., Dinan, T. G. & Cryan, J. F. (2015). A natural solution for obesity: Bioactives for the prevention and treatment of weight gain. A review. *Nutritional Neuroscience, 18*(2), 49–65.

91   Mohamed, G. A., Ibrahim, S. R., Elkhayat, E. S. & El Dine, R. S. (2014). Natural anti-obesity agents. *Bulletin of Faculty of Pharmacy, Cairo University, 52*(2), 269–284.
92   Bo-Linn, G. W., Ana, C. A. S., Morawski, S. G. & Fordtran, J. S. (1982). Starch blockers—Their effect on calorie absorption from a high-starch meal. *New England Journal of Medicine, 307*(23), 1413–1416.
93   Eckerson, J. M. (2015). Weight loss nutritional supplements. In M. Greenwood, M. Cooke, T. Ziegenfuss, D. S. Kalman & J. Antonio (eds), *Nutritional Supplements in Sports and Exercise: Second Edition* (pp. 159–185). London: Springer International. DOI: 10.1007/978-3-319-18230-8-8
94   Dziki, D., Gawlik-Dziki, U., Pecio, Ł., Różyło, R., Świeca, M., Krzykowski, A. & Rudy, S. (2015). Ground green coffee beans as a functional food supplement: Preliminary study. *LWT–Food Science and Technology, 63*(1), 691–699.
95   Flanagan, J., Bily, A., Rolland, Y. & Roller, M. (2014). Lipolytic activity of Svetol®, a decaffeinated green coffee bean extract. *Phytotherapy Research, 28*(6), 946–948.
96   Buchanan, R. & Beckett, R. D. (2013). Green coffee for pharmacological weight loss. *Journal of Evidence-Based Complementary & Alternative Medicine*, 2156587213496818.
97   Sarriá, B., Martínez-López, S., Mateos, R. & Bravo-Clemente, L. (2016). Long-term consumption of a green/roasted coffee blend positively affects glucose metabolism and insulin resistance in humans. *Food Research International, 89*, 1023–1028.
98   Chokshi, D. (2006). Toxicity studies of Blockal, a dietary supplement containing Phase 2 Starch Neutralizer (Phase 2), a standardized extract of the common white kidney bean (*Phaseolus vulgaris*). *International Journal of Toxicology, 25*(5), 361–371.
99   Udani, J. & Singh, B. B. (2007). Blocking carbohydrate absorption and weight loss: a clinical trial using a proprietary fractionated white bean extract. *Alternative Therapies in Health and Medicine, 13*(4), 32–37.
100   Preuss, H. G. (2009). Bean amylase inhibitor and other carbohydrate absorption blockers: Effects on diabesity and general health. *Journal of the American College of Nutrition, 28*(3), 266–276.
101   Budak, N. H., Aykin, E., Seydim, A. C., Greene, A. K. & Guzel-Seydim, Z. B. (2014). Functional properties of vinegar. *Journal of Food Science, 79*(5), R757–R764.
102   Nazıroğlu, M., Güler, M., Özgül, C., Saydam, G., Küçükayaz, M. & Sözbir, E. (2014). Apple cider vinegar modulates serum lipid profile, erythrocyte, kidney, and liver membrane oxidative stress in ovariectomized mice fed high cholesterol. *The Journal of Membrane Biology, 247*(8), 667–673.
103   Petsiou, E. I., Mitrou, P. I., Raptis, S. A., & Dimitriadis, G. D. (2014). Effect and mechanisms of action of vinegar on glucose metabolism, lipid profile, and body weight. *Nutrition Reviews, 72*(10), 651–661.
104   Darzi, J., Frost, G. S., Montaser, R., Yap, J. & Robertson, M. D. (2014). Influence of the tolerability of vinegar as an oral source of short-chain fatty acids on appetite control and food intake. *International Journal of Obesity, 38*(5), 675–681.
105   Beheshti, Z., Chan, Y. H., Nia, H. S., Hajihosseini, F., Nazari, R. & Shaabani, M. (2012). Influence of apple cider vinegar on blood lipids. *Life Science Journal, 9*(4), 2431–2440.
106   Jeukendrup, A. E. & Randell, R. (2011). Fat burners: Nutrition supplements that increase fat metabolism. *Obesity Reviews, 12*(10), 841–851.
107   Hawley, J. A. (1998). Fat burning during exercise: Can ergogenics change the balance? *The Physician and Sportsmedicine, 26*(9), 56–68.
108   Radha Krishna, Y., Mittal, V., Grewal, P., Fiel, M. I. & Schiano, T. (2011). Acute liver failure caused by "fat burners" and dietary supplements: A case report and literature review. *Canadian Journal of Gastroenterology and Hepatology, 25*(3), 157–160.
109   Dwyer, J. T., Allison, D. B. & Coates, P. M. (2005). Dietary supplements in weight reduction. *Journal of the American Dietetic Association, 105*(5), 80–86.
110   Huntington, M. K. & Shewmake, R. A. (2010). Weight-loss supplements: What is the evidence? *South Dakota Medicine, 63*(6), 205–207.

111 Pariza, M. W. (2004). Perspective on the safety and effectiveness of conjugated linoleic acid. *The American Journal of Clinical Nutrition, 79*(6), 1132S–1136S.

112 DeLany, J. P., Blohm, F., Truett, A. A., Scimeca, J. A. & West, D. B. (1999). Conjugated linoleic acid rapidly reduces body fat content in mice without affecting energy intake. *American Journal of Physiology–Regulatory, Integrative and Comparative Physiology, 276*(4), R1172–R1179.

113 Kamphuis, M. M. J. W., Lejeune, M. P. G. M., Saris, W. H. M. & Westerterp-Plantenga, M. S. (2003). The effect of conjugated linoleic acid supplementation after weight loss on body weight regain, body composition, and resting metabolic rate in overweight subjects. *International Journal of Obesity, 27*(7), 840–847.

114 Cornish, S. M., McBreairty, L., Chilibeck, P. D. & Zello, G. A. (2016). Fat metabolism during exercise and dietary interventions for enhancing fat metabolism and athletic performance. *Handbook of Lipids in Human Function: Fatty Acids*, 499.

115 Barone, R., Macaluso, F., Catanese, P., Gammazza, A. M., Rizzuto, L., Marozzi, P., Giudice, G. L., Stampone, T., Cappello, F., Morici, G. & Zummo, G. (2013). Endurance exercise and conjugated linoleic acid (CLA) supplementation up-regulate CYP17A1 and stimulate testosterone biosynthesis. *PloS One, 8*(11), e79686.

116 Lehnen, T. E., da Silva, M. R., Camacho, A., Marcadenti, A. & Lehnen, A. M. (2015). A review on effects of conjugated linoleic fatty acid (CLA) upon body composition and energetic metabolism. *Journal of the International Society of Sports Nutrition, 12*(1), 36.

117 Kamphuis, M. M. J. W., Lejeune, M. P. G. M., Saris, W. H. M. & Westerterp-Plantenga, M. S. (2003). Effect of conjugated linoleic acid supplementation after weight loss on appetite and food intake in overweight subjects. *European Journal of Clinical Nutrition, 57*(10), 1268–1274.

118 Pariza, M. W. (2004). Perspective on the safety and effectiveness of conjugated linoleic acid. *The American Journal of Clinical Nutrition, 79*(6), 1132S–1136S.

119 Chen, I. J., Liu, C. Y., Chiu, J. P. & Hsu, C. H. (2016). Therapeutic effect of high-dose green tea extract on weight reduction: A randomized, double-blind, placebo-controlled clinical trial. *Clinical Nutrition, 35*(3), 592–599.

120 Janssens, P. L., Hursel, R., & Westerterp-Plantenga, M. S. (2015). Long-term green tea extract supplementation does not affect fat absorption, resting energy expenditure, and body composition in adults. *The Journal of Nutrition*, jn-114.

121 Janssens, P. L., Hursel, R. & Westerterp-Plantenga, M. S. (2015). Long-term green tea extract supplementation does not affect fat absorption, resting energy expenditure, and body composition in adults. *The Journal of Nutrition, 145*(5), 864–870.

122 Mielgo-Ayuso, J., Barrenechea, L., Alcorta, P., Larrarte, E., Margareto, J. & Labayen, I. (2014). Effects of dietary supplementation with epigallocatechin-3-gallate on weight loss, energy homeostasis, cardiometabolic risk factors and liver function in obese women: Randomised, double-blind, placebo-controlled clinical trial. *British Journal of Nutrition, 111*(7), 1263–1271.

123 Patel, S. S., Beer, S., Kearney, D. L., Phillips, G. & Carter, B. A. (2013). Green tea extract: A potential cause of acute liver failure. *World Journal of Gastroenterol, 19*(31), 5174–5177.

124 Farghali, H., Canova, N. K. & Lekiæ, N. (2013). Resveratrol and related compounds as antioxidants with an allosteric mechanism of action in epigenetic drug targets. *Physiological Research, 62*(1), 1–13.

125 Ristow, M. (2014). Unraveling the truth about antioxidants: mitohormesis explains ROS-induced health benefits. *Nature Medicine, 20*(7), 709–711.

126 Ristow, M., Zarse, K., Oberbach, A., Klöting, N., Birringer, M., Kiehntopf, M., Stumvoll, M., Kahn, C. R. & Blüher, M. (2009). Antioxidants prevent health-promoting effects of physical exercise in humans. *Proceedings of the National Academy of Sciences, 106*(21), 8665–8670.

127 Pingitore, A., Lima, G. P. P., Mastorci, F., Quinones, A., Iervasi, G. & Vassalle, C. (2015). Exercise and oxidative stress: Potential effects of antioxidant dietary strategies in sports. *Nutrition, 31*(7), 916–922.

128 Braakhuis, A. J. & Hopkins, W. G. (2015). Impact of dietary antioxidants on sport performance: A review. *Sports Medicine*, *45*(7), 939–955.

129 Braakhuis, A. J., Hopkins, W. G. & Lowe, T. E. (2014). Effects of dietary antioxidants on training and performance in female runners. *European Journal of Sport Science*, *14*(2), 160–168.

130 Somerville, V., Bringans, C. & Braakhuis, A. (2017). Polyphenols and performance: A systematic review and meta-analysis. *Sports Medicine*, *47*(8), 1–11.

131 McFarlin, B. K., Venable, A. S., Henning, A. L., Sampson, J. N. B., Pennel, K., Vingren, J. L. & Hill, D. W. (2016). Reduced inflammatory and muscle damage biomarkers following oral supplementation with bioavailable curcumin. *BBA Clinical*, *5*, 72–78.

132 Bar-Sela, G., Epelbaum, R. & Schaffer, M. (2010). Curcumin as an anti-cancer agent: Review of the gap between basic and clinical applications. *Current Medicinal Chemistry*, *17*(3), 190–197; Devassy, J. G., Nwachukwu, I. D. & Jones, P. J. (2015). Curcumin and cancer: Barriers to obtaining a health claim. *Nutrition Reviews*, *73*(3), 155–165.

133 Akram, M., Shahab-Uddin, A. A., Usmanghani, K., Hannan, A., Mohiuddin, E. & Asif, M. (2010). Curcuma longa and curcumin: A review article. *Romanian Journal of Biology—Plant Biology*, *55*(2), 65–70.

134 Delecroix, B., Abaïdia, A. E., Leduc, C., Dawson, B. & Dupont, G. (2017). Curcumin and Piperine supplementation and recovery following exercise induced muscle samage: A randomized controlled trial. *Journal of Sports Science & Medicine*, *16*(1), 147.

135 Nicol, L. M., Rowlands, D. S., Fazakerly, R. & Kellett, J. (2015). Curcumin supplementation likely attenuates delayed onset muscle soreness (DOMS). *European Journal of Applied Physiology*, *115*(8), 1769–1777.

136 Tanabe, Y., Maeda, S., Akazawa, N., Zempo-Miyaki, A., Choi, Y., Ra, S. G., Imaizumi, A., Otsuka, Y. & Nosaka, K. (2015). Attenuation of indirect markers of eccentric exercise-induced muscle damage by curcumin. *European Journal of Applied Physiology*, *115*(9), 1949–1957.

137 Tong, H., Rappold, A. G., Caughey, M., Hinderliter, A. L., Bassett, M., Montilla, T., Case, M. W., Berntsen, J., Bromberg, P. A., Cascio, W. E. & Diaz-Sanchez, D., 2015. Dietary supplementation with olive oil or fish oil and vascular effects of concentrated ambient particulate matter exposure in human volunteers. *Environmental Health Perspectives*, *123*(11), 1173–1179.

138 Jakeman, J. R., Lambrick, D. M., Wooley, B., Babraj, J. A. & Faulkner, J. A. (2017). Effect of an acute dose of omega-3 fish oil following exercise-induced muscle damage. *European Journal of Applied Physiology*, *117*(3), 575–582.

139 Gray, P., Chappell, A., Jenkinson, A. M., Thies, F. & Gray, S. R. (2014). Fish oil supplementation reduces markers of oxidative stress but not muscle soreness after eccentric exercise. *International Journal of Sport Nutrition and Exercise Metabolism*, *24*(2), 206–214; Pearson, S. J., Johnson, T. & Robins, A. (2014). Fish oil supplementation, resting blood flow and markers of cellular metabolism during incremental exercise. *International Journal for Vitamin and Nutrition Research*, *84*(1–2), 18–26.

140 McGlory, C., Wardle, S. L., Macnaughton, L. S., Witard, O. C., Scott, F., Dick, J., Bell, J. G., Phillips, S. M., Galloway, S. D., Hamilton, D. L. & Tipton, K. D. (2016). Fish oil supplementation suppresses resistance exercise and feeding-induced increases in anabolic signaling without affecting myofibrillar protein synthesis in young men. *Physiological Reports*, *4*(6), e12715.

141 Bolland, M. J., Grey, A., Gamble, G. D. & Reid, I. R. (2014). The effect of vitamin D supplementation on skeletal, vascular, or cancer outcomes: A trial sequential meta-analysis. *The Lancet Diabetes & Endocrinology*, *2*(4), 307–320; Cameron-Smith, D., Albert, B. B. & Cutfield, W. S. (2015). Fishing for answers: is oxidation of fish oil supplements a problem? *Journal of Nutritional Science*, *4*, e36.

142 Bolland, M. J., Grey, A., Gamble, G. D. & Reid, I. R. (2014). The effect of vitamin D supplementation on skeletal, vascular, or cancer outcomes: A trial sequential meta-analysis. *The Lancet Diabetes & Endocrinology*, *2*(4), 307–320.

143 Lombardi, G., Vitale, J. A., Logoluso, S., Logoluso, G., Cocco, N., Cocco, G., Cocco, A. & Banfi, G. (2017). Circannual rhythm of plasmatic vitamin D levels and the association with markers of psychophysical stress in a cohort of Italian professional soccer players. *Chronobiology International*, *34*(4), 471–479.

144 Close, G. L., Russell, J., Cobley, J. N., Owens, D. J., Wilson, G., Gregson, W., Fraser, W. D. & Morton, J. P. (2013). Assessment of vitamin D concentration in non-supplemented professional athletes and healthy adults during the winter months in the UK: Implications for skeletal muscle function. *Journal of Sports Sciences*, *31*(4), 344–353.

145 Autier, P., Boniol, M., Pizot, C. & Mullie, P. (2014). Vitamin D status and ill health: A systematic review. *The Lancet Diabetes & Endocrinology*, *2*(1), 76–89; Bolland, M. J., Grey, A., Gamble, G. D. & Reid, I. R. (2014). The effect of vitamin D supplementation on skeletal, vascular, or cancer outcomes: A trial sequential meta-analysis. *The Lancet Diabetes & Endocrinology*, *2*(4), 307–320; Reid, I. R., Bolland, M. J. & Grey, A. (2014). Effects of vitamin D supplements on bone mineral density: A systematic review and meta-analysis. *The Lancet*, *383*(9912), 146–155.

146 Mattison, J. A., Wang, M., Bernier, M., Zhang, J., Park, S. S., Maudsley, S., An, S. S., Santhanam, L., Martin, B., Faulkner, S. & Morrell, C. (2014). Resveratrol prevents high fat/sucrose diet-induced central arterial wall inflammation and stiffening in nonhuman primates. *Cell Metabolism*, *20*(1), 183–190.

147 Bureau, G., Longpré, F. & Martinoli, M. G. (2008). Resveratrol and quercetin, two natural polyphenols, reduce apoptotic neuronal cell death induced by neuro-inflammation. *Journal of Neuroscience Research*, *86*(2), 403–410.

148 Laupheimer, M. W., Perry, M., Benton, S., Malliaras, P. & Maffulli, N. (2014). Resveratrol exerts no effect on inflammatory response and delayed onset muscle soreness after a marathon in male athletes: A randomised, double-blind, placebo-controlled pilot feasibility study. *Translational Medicine@ UniSa*, *10*, 38–42.

149 Gliemann, L., Schmidt, J. F., Olesen, J., Biensø, R. S., Peronard, S. L., Grandjean, S. U., Mortensen, S. P., Nyberg, M., Bangsbo, J., Pilegaard, H. & Hellsten, Y. (2013). Resveratrol blunts the positive effects of exercise training on cardiovascular health in aged men. *The Journal of Physiology*, *591*(20), 5047–5059.

150 Liu, K., Zhou, R., Wang, B. & Mi, M. T. (2014). Effect of resveratrol on glucose control and insulin sensitivity: A meta-analysis of 11 randomized controlled trials. *The American Journal of Clinical Nutrition*, *99*(6), 1510–1519.

151 Macedo, R. C. S., Vieira, A., Marin, D. P. & Otton, R. (2015). Effects of chronic resveratrol supplementation in military firefighters undergo a physical fitness test— A placebo-controlled, double blind study. *Chemico-biological Interactions*, *227*, 89–95.

152 Aoi, W., Naito, Y. & Yoshikawa, T. (2006). Exercise and functional foods. *Nutrition Journal*, *5*(1), 15–23.

153 Hespel, P., Maughan, R. J. & Greenhaff, P. L. (2006). Dietary supplements for football. *Journal of Sports Sciences*, *24*(7), 749–761.

154 Bascoul-Colombo, C., Garaiova, I., Plummer, S. F., Harwood, J. L., Caterson, B. & Hughes, C. E. (2016). Glucosamine hydrochloride but not chondroitin sulfate prevents cartilage degradation and inflammation induced by interleukin-1α in bovine cartilage explants. *Cartilage*, *7*(1), 70–81.

155 Braham, R., Dawson, B. & Goodman, C. (2003). The effect of glucosamine supplementation on people experiencing regular knee pain. *British Journal of Sports Medicine*, *37*(1), 45–49.

156 Vad, V., Hong, H. M., Zazzali, M., Agi, N. & Basrai, D. (2002). Exercise recommendations in athletes with early osteoarthritis of the knee. *Sports Medicine*, *32*(11), 729–739.

157 See, for example, www.health.harvard.edu/staying-healthy/listing_of_vitamins

158 McClung, J. P., Gaffney-Stomberg, E. & Lee, J. J. (2014). Female athletes: A population at risk of vitamin and mineral deficiencies affecting health and performance. *Journal of Trace Elements in Medicine and Biology*, *28*(4), 388–392.

159   Brisswalter, J. & Louis, J. (2014). Vitamin supplementation benefits in master athletes. *Sports Medicine*, *44*(3), 311–318.

160   Wiens, K., Erdman, K. A., Stadnyk, M. & Parnell, J. A. (2014). Dietary supplement usage, motivation, and education in young Canadian athletes. *International Journal of Sport Nutrition and Exercise Metabolism*, *24*(6), 613–622.

161   Guallar, E., Stranges, S., Mulrow, C., Appel, L. J. & Miller, E. R. (2013). Enough is enough: Stop wasting money on vitamin and mineral supplements. *Annals of Internal Medicine*, *159*(12), 850–851; Volpe, S. L. & Nguyen, H. (2013). Vitamins, minerals, and sport performance. *The Encyclopaedia of Sports Medicine: An IOC Medical Commission Publication*, *19*, 215–228.

162   Wildman, R. E. (ed.). (2016). *Handbook of nutraceuticals and functional foods*. Boca Raton, FL: CRC Press.

163   Brennan, R., Van Hout, M. C. & Wells, J. (2013). Heuristics of human enhancement risk: A little chemical help? *International Journal of Health Promotion and Education*, *51*(4), 212–227.

164   Brennan, R., Wells, J. S. & Van Hout, M. C. (2016). The injecting use of image and performance-enhancing drugs (IPED) in the general population: A systematic review. *Health & Social Care in the Community*, doi:10.1111/hsc.12326.

165   Figueiredo, V. C. & Silva, P. R. P. D. (2014). Cosmetic Doping—When anabolic-androgenic steroids are not enough. *Substance Use & Misuse*, *49*(9), 1163–1167.

166   Zamora, A. C., Collard, H. R., Barrera, L., Mendoza, F., Webb, W. R. & Carrillo, G. (2009). Silicone injection causing acute pneumonitis: A case series. *Lung*, *187*(4), 241–244.

167   Kannan, R. Y., Sankar, T. K. & Ward, D. J. (2010). The disaster of DIY breast augmentation. *Journal of Plastic, Reconstructive & Aesthetic Surgery*, *63*(1), e100–e101.

168   Restrepo, C. S., Artunduaga, M., Carrillo, J. A., Rivera, A. L., Ojeda, P., Martinez-Jimenez, S., Manzano, A. C. & Rossi, S. E. (2009). Silicone pulmonary embolism: Report of 10 cases and review of the literature. *Journal of Computer Assisted Tomography*, *33*(2), 233–237.

169   Kannan, R. Y., Sankar, T. K. & Ward, D. J. (2010). The disaster of DIY breast augmentation. *Journal of Plastic, Reconstructive & Aesthetic Surgery*, *63*(1), e100–e101.

170   Berkowitz, D. (2017). *Botox Nation: Changing the Face of America*. New York: NYU Press.

171   Verma, A., Srivastava, S., Kharbanda, S., Priyadarshini, J. & Gupta, A. (2015). Botox: Tales beyond beauty. *Journal of Evolution of Medical and Dental Sciences–JEMDS*, *4*(69), 12068–12074.

172   Lewis, W. (2014). The rise in black market aesthetic products. *Prime*, *4*(4), 12–17.

173   Liang, B. A., Mackey, T. K. & Lovett, K. (2012). Emerging dangers from direct botulinum access and use. *Journal of Homeland Security Emergency Management*, *9*(1), doi.org/10.1515/1547-7355.1973.

174   Toy, B. R. & Frank, P. J. (2003). Review outbreak of mycobacterium abscessus infection after soft tissue augmentation. *Dermatological Surgery*, *29*(9), 971–973.

175   Coté, T. R., Mohan, A. K., Polder, J. A., Walton, M. K. & Braun, M. M. (2005). Botulinum toxin type A injections: Adverse events reported to the US Food and Drug Administration in therapeutic and cosmetic cases. *Journal of the American Academy of Dermatology*, *53*(3), 407–415.

176   Pupka, A., Sikora, J., Mauricz, J., Cios, D. & Płonek, T. (2008). The usage of synthol in the body building. *Polimery w Medycynie*, *39*(1), 63–65.

177   Smith, A. C. & Stewart, B. (2012). Body conceptions and virtual ethnopharmacology in an online bodybuilding community. *Performance Enhancement & Health*, *1*(1), 35–38.

178   Schäfer, C. N., Hvolris, J., Karlsmark, T. & Plambech, M. (2012). Muscle enhancement using intramuscular injections of oil in bodybuilding: Review on epidemiology, complications, clinical evaluation and treatment. *European Surgery*, *44*(2), 109–115.

179   Hall, M., Grogan, S. & Gough, B. (2016). Bodybuilders' accounts of synthol use: The construction of lay expertise online. *Journal of Health Psychology*, *21*(9), 1939–1948.

180   Banke, I. J., Prodinger, P. M., Waldt, S., Weirich, G., Holzapfel, B. M., Gradinger, R. & Rechl, H. (2012). Irreversible muscle damage in bodybuilding due to long-term intramuscular oil injection. *International Journal of Sports Medicine*, *33*(10), 829–834.

181   Ghandourah, S., Hofer, M. J., Kießling, A., El-Zayat, B. & Schofer, M. D. (2012). Painful muscle fibrosis following synthol injections in a bodybuilder: A case report. *Journal of Medical Case Reports*, *6*(1), 248.

182   Banke, I. J., Prodinger, P. M., Waldt, S., Weirich, G., Holzapfel, B. M., Gradinger, R. & Rechl, H. (2012). Irreversible muscle damage in bodybuilding due to long-term intramuscular oil injection. *International Journal of Sports Medicine*, *33*(10), 829–834.

183   Herr, A., Rehmert, G., Kunde, K., Gust, R. & Gries, A. (2002). A thirty-year old bodybuilder with septic shock and ARDS from abuse of anabolic steroids. *Der Anaesthesist*, *51*(7), 557–563.

184   Petersen, M. L., Colville-Ebeling, B., Jensen, T. H. L. & Hougen, H. P. (2015). Intramuscular injection of "Site Enhancement Oil": Forensic considerations. *The American Journal of Forensic Medicine and Pathology*, *36*(2), 53–55.

185   Petersen, M. L., Colville-Ebeling, B., Jensen, T. H. L. & Hougen, H. P. (2015). Intramuscular injection of "Site Enhancement Oil": Forensic considerations. *The American Journal of Forensic Medicine and Pathology*, *36*(2), 53–55.

186   Evans-Brown, M., McVeigh, J., Perkins, C. & Bellis, M. A. (2012). *Human enhancement drugs: The emerging challenges to public health*. Liverpool, UK: Public Health Observatories in England.

187   Langan, E. A., Nie, Z. & Rhodes, L. E. (2010). Melanotropic peptides: More than just "Barbie drugs" and "sun-tan jabs"? *British Journal of Dermatology*, *163*(3), 451–455.

188   Mahiques-Santos, L. 2012. Melanotan. *Actas Dermo-Sifiliograficas*, *103*, 257–259.

189   Brennan, R., Wells, J. G. & Van Hout, M. C. (2014). An unhealthy glow? A review of melanotan use and associated clinical outcomes. *Performance Enhancement & Health*, *3*(2), 78–92.

190   Ferrándiz-Pulido, C., Fernández-Figueras, M. T., Quer, A. & Ferrándiz, C. (2011). An eruptive pigmented lesion after melanotan injection. *Clinical and Experimental Dermatology*, *36*(7), 801–802.

191   Van Hout, M. C. & Brennan, R. (2014). An in-depth case examination of an exotic dancer's experience of melanotan. *International Journal of Drug Policy*, *25*(3), 444–450.

192   Van Hout, M. C. (2014). SMART: An Internet study of users' experiences of synthetic tanning. *Performance Enhancement & Health*, *3*(1), 3–14.

193   Barceloux, D. G. & Palmer, R. B. (2013). Anabolic-androgenic steroids. *Dis Mon*, *59*(6), 226–248.

194   Papaloucas, M., Kyriazi, K. & Kouloulias, V. (2015). Pheromones: A new ergogenic aid in sport? *International Journal of Sports Physiology and Performance*, *10*(7), 939–940.

195   Thevis, M. & Schänzer, W. (2010). Synthetic anabolic agents: steroids and nonsteroidal selective androgen receptor modulators. In D. Thieme & P. Hemmersbach (eds), *Doping in Sports: Biochemical Principles, Effects and Analysis* (pp. 99–126). Berlin: Springer.

196   Zhi, L. & Martinborough, E. (2001). Selective androgen receptor modulators (SARMs). *Annual Reports in Medicinal Chemistry*, *36*, 169–180.

197   Thevis, M. & Schänzer, W. (2010). Synthetic anabolic agents: steroids and nonsteroidal selective androgen receptor modulators. In D. Thieme & P. Hemmersbach (eds), *Doping in Sports: Biochemical Principles, Effects and Analysis* (pp. 99–126). Berlin: Springer.

198   Christou, M. A., Christou, P. A., Markozannes, G., Tsatsoulis, A., Mastorakos, G. & Tigas, S. (2017). Effects of anabolic androgenic steroids on the reproductive system of athletes and recreational users: A systematic review and meta-analysis. *Sports Medicine*, 1–15; Nieschlag, E. & Vorona, E. (2015). Mechanisms in endocrinology: Medical consequences of doping with anabolic androgenic steroids: effects on reproductive functions. *European Journal of Endocrinology*, *173*(2), R47–R58.

199 Kanayama, G., Hudson, J. I., DeLuca, J., Isaacs, S., Baggish, A., Weiner, R., Bhasin, S. & Pope, H. G. (2015). Prolonged hypogonadism in males following withdrawal from anabolic–androgenic steroids: An under-recognized problem. *Addiction*, *110*(5), 823–831.

200 Pope, H. G., Kanayama, G., Athey, A., Ryan, E., Hudson, J. I. & Baggish, A. (2014). The lifetime prevalence of anabolic-androgenic steroid use and dependence in Americans: Current best estimates. *The American Journal on Addictions*, *23*(4), 371–377.

201 Bahrke, M. S., Yesalis, C. E. & Wright, J. E. (1996). Psychological and behavioural effects of endogenous testosterone and anabolic-androgenic steroids. *Sports Medicine*, *22*(6), 367–390.

202 Elashoff, J. D., Jacknow, A. D., Shain, S. G. & Braunstein, G. D. (1991). Effects of anabolic–androgenic steroids on muscular strength. *Annals of Internal Medicine*, *115*(5), 387–393; Friedl, K. E. (2015). US Army research on pharmacological enhancement of soldier performance: Stimulants, anabolic hormones, and blood doping. *The Journal of Strength & Conditioning Research*, *29*, S71–S76; Gomes, F. G. N., Fernandes, J., Campos, D. V., Cassilhas, R. C., Viana, G. M., D'Almeida, V., de Moraes Rêgo, M. K., Buainain, P. I., Cavalheiro, E. A. & Arida, R. M. (2014). The beneficial effects of strength exercise on hippocampal cell proliferation and apoptotic signaling is impaired by anabolic androgenic steroids. *Psychoneuroendocrinology*, *50*, 106–117; Hassan, A. & Kamal, M. M. (2013). Effect of exercise training and anabolic androgenic steroids on hemodynamics, glycogen content, angiogenesis and apoptosis of cardiac muscle in adult male rats. *International Journal of Health Sciences*, *7*(1), 47–60; Yu, J. G., Bonnerud, P., Eriksson, A., Stål, P. S., Tegner, Y. & Malm, C. (2014). Effects of long term supplementation of anabolic androgen steroids on human skeletal muscle. *PloS one*, *9*(9), e105330.

203 El Osta, R., Almont, T., Diligent, C., Hubert, N., Eschwège, P. & Hubert, J. (2016). Anabolic steroids abuse and male infertility. *Basic and Clinical Andrology*, *26*(1), 2; Frati, P., P Busardo, F., Cipolloni, L., De Dominicis, E. & Fineschi, V. (2015). Anabolic androgenic steroid (AAS) related deaths: Autoptic, histopathological and toxicological findings. *Current Neuropharmacology*, *13*(1), 146–159; Hildebrandt, T., Langenbucher, J. W., Flores, A., Harty, S. & Berlin, H. A. (2014). The influence of age of onset and acute anabolic steroid exposure on cognitive performance, impulsivity, and aggression in men. *Psychology of Addictive Behaviors*, *28*(4), 1096; Kanayama, G., DeLuca, J., Meehan III, W. P., Hudson, J. I., Isaacs, S., Baggish, A., Weiner, R., Micheli, L. & Pope Jr, H. G. (2015). Ruptured tendons in anabolic-androgenic steroid users: a cross-sectional cohort study. *The American Journal of Sports Medicine*, *43*(11), 2638–2644; Kanayama, G., Kean, J., Hudson, J. I. & Pope, H. G. (2013). Cognitive deficits in long-term anabolic-androgenic steroid users. *Drug and Alcohol Dependence*, *130*(1), 208–214; Kaufman, M. J., Janes, A. C., Hudson, J. I., Brennan, B. P., Kanayama, G., Kerrigan, A. R., Jensen, J. E. & Pope, H. G. (2015). Brain and cognition abnormalities in long-term anabolic–androgenic steroid users. *Drug and Alcohol Dependence*, *152*, 47–56; Lundholm, L., Frisell, T., Lichtenstein, P. & Långström, N. (2015). Anabolic androgenic steroids and violent offending: Confounding by polysubstance abuse among 10 365 general population men. *Addiction*, *110*(1), 100–108; Nieschlag, E. & Vorona, E. (2015). Doping with anabolic androgenic steroids (AAS): Adverse effects on non-reproductive organs and functions. *Reviews in Endocrine and Metabolic Disorders*, *16*(3), 199–211; Onakomaiya, M. M. & Henderson, L. P. (2016). Mad men, women and steroid cocktails: A review of the impact of sex and other factors on anabolic androgenic steroids effects on affective behaviors. *Psychopharmacology*, *233*(4), 549–569; Nieschlag, E. & Vorona, E. (2015). Doping with anabolic androgenic steroids (AAS): Adverse effects on non-reproductive organs and functions. *Reviews in Endocrine and Metabolic Disorders*, *16*(3), 199–211; Pereira dos Santos, M. A., Coutinho de Oliveira, C. V. & Silva, A. S. (2014). Adverse cardiovascular effects from the use of anabolic-androgenic steroids as ergogenic resources. *Substance Use & Misuse*, *49*(9), 1132–1137; Pope, H. G. & Katz, D. L. (1994). Psychiatric and medical effects of anabolic-

androgenic steroid use: A controlled study of 160 athletes. *Archives of General Psychiatry*, *51*(5), 375–382; van Amsterdam, J. & Hartgens, F. (2014). Acute and chronic adverse reaction of anabolic–androgenic steroids. *Adverse Drug Reaction Bulletin*, *288*(1), 1111–1114; Zahnow, R., McVeigh, J., Ferris, J. & Winstock, A. (2017). Adverse effects, health service engagement, and service satisfaction among anabolic androgenic steroid users. *Contemporary Drug Problems*, *44*(1), 69–83.

204 Darke, S., Torok, M. & Duflou, J. (2014). Sudden or unnatural deaths involving anabolic-androgenic steroids. *Journal of Forensic Sciences*, *59*(4), 1025–1028.

205 Kanayama, G., Hudson, J. I., DeLuca, J., Isaacs, S., Baggish, A., Weiner, R., Bhasin, S. & Pope, H. G. (2015). Prolonged hypogonadism in males following withdrawal from anabolic–androgenic steroids: An under-recognized problem. *Addiction*, *110*(5), 823–831; Rasmussen, J. J., Selmer, C., Østergren, P. B., Pedersen, K. B., Schou, M., Gustafsson, F., Faber, J., Juul, A. & Kistorp, C. (2016). Former abusers of anabolic androgenic steroids exhibit decreased testosterone levels and hypogonadal symptoms years after cessation: A case-control study. *PloS one*, *11*(8), e0161208.

206 LaBotz, M. & Griesemer, B. A. (2016). Use of performance-enhancing substances. *Pediatrics*, e20161300; Patel, D. R. & Greydanus, D. E. (2015). Adolescent athletes and sports doping. *International Public Health Journal*, *7*(2), 221; White, N. D. & Noeun, J. (2016). Performance-enhancing drug use in adolescence. *American Journal of Lifestyle Medicine*, 1559827616680593.

207 Thevis, M., Thomas, A. & Schänzer, W. (2014). Detecting peptidic drugs, drug candidates and analogs in sports doping: Current status and future directions. *Expert Review of Proteomics*, *11*(6), 663–673.

208 Thevis, M., Kuuranne, T., Geyer, H. & Schänzer, W. (2017). Annual banned-substance review: analytical approaches in human sports drug testing. *Drug Testing and Analysis*, *9*(1), 6–29.

209 Birzniece, V. (2015). Doping in sport: effects, harm and misconceptions. *Internal Medicine Journal*, *45*(3), 239–248.

210 Salamin, O., Kuuranne, T., Saugy, M. & Leuenberger, N. (2017). Erythropoietin as a performance-enhancing drug: Its mechanistic basis, detection, and potential adverse effects. *Molecular and Cellular Endocrinology*. doi.org/10.1016/j.mce.2017.01.033

211 Adamson, J. W. & Vapnek, D. (1991). Recombinant erythropoietin to improve athletic performance. *New England Journal of Medicine*, *324*(10), 698–699; Caillaud, C., Connes, P., Saad, H. B. & Mercier, J. (2015). Erythropoietin enhances whole body lipid oxidation during prolonged exercise in humans. *Journal of Physiology and Biochemistry*, *71*(1), 9–16; Guadalupe-Grau, A., Plenge, U., Helbo, S., Kristensen, M., Andersen, P. R., Fago, A., Belhage, B., Dela, F. & Helge, J. W. (2015). Effects of an 8-weeks erythropoietin treatment on mitochondrial and whole body fat oxidation capacity during exercise in healthy males. *Journal of Sports Sciences*, *33*(6), 570–578; La Gerche, A. & Brosnan, M. J. (2017). Cardiovascular effects of performance-enhancing drugs. *Circulation*, *135*(1), 89–99; Miskowiak, K. W., Macoveanu, J., Vinberg, M., Assentoft, E., Randers, L., Harmer, C. J., Ehrenreich, H., Paulson, O. B., Knudsen, G. M., Siebner, H. R. & Kessing, L. V. (2016). Effects of erythropoietin on memory-relevant neurocircuitry activity and recall in mood disorders. *Acta Psychiatrica Scandinavica*, *134*(3), 249–259; Miskowiak, K. W., Vinberg, M., Macoveanu, J., Ehrenreich, H., Køster, N., Inkster, B., Paulson, O. B., Kessing, L. V., Skimminge, A. & Siebner, H. R. (2015). Effects of erythropoietin on hippocampal volume and memory in mood disorders. *Biological Psychiatry*, *78*(4), 270–277; Salamin, O., Kuuranne, T., Saugy, M. & Leuenberger, N. (2017). Erythropoietin as a performance-enhancing drug: Its mechanistic basis, detection, and potential adverse effects. *Molecular and Cellular Endocrinology*, Jan 22; Smith, K. J., Bleyer, A. J., Little, W. C. & Sane, D. C. (2003). The cardiovascular effects of erythropoietin. *Cardiovascular Research*, *59*(3), 538–548; Thomsen, J. J., Rentsch, R. L., Robach, P., Calbet, J. A. L., Boushel, R., Rasmussen, P., Juel, C. & Lundby, C. (2007). Prolonged administration of

recombinant human erythropoietin increases submaximal performance more than maximal aerobic capacity. *European Journal of Applied Physiology*, *101*(4), 481–486.

212 Baron, D. A., Reardon, C. L. & Baron, S. H. (2013). Doping in sport. *Clinical Sports Psychiatry: An International Perspective*, 21–32; Birzniece, V. (2015). Doping in sport: effects, harm and misconceptions. *Internal Medicine Journal*, *45*(3), 239–248; Breda, E., Benders, J. & Kuipers, H. (2014). Little soldiers in their cardboard cells. *British Journal of Clinical Pharmacology*, 77(3), 580–581; Cernaro, V., Lacquaniti, A., Buemi, A., Lupica, R. & Buemi, M. (2014). Does erythropoietin always win? *Current Medicinal Chemistry*, *21*(7), 849–854; Citartan, M., Gopinath, S. C., Chen, Y., Lakshmipriya, T. & Tang, T. H. (2015). Monitoring recombinant human erythropoietin abuse among athletes. *Biosensors and Bioelectronics*, *63*, 86–98; Reardon, C. L. & Creado, S. (2014). Drug abuse in athletes. *Substance Abuse and Rehabilitation*, *5*, 95–105; Tokish, J. M., Kocher, M. S. & Hawkins, R. J. (2004). Ergogenic aids: A review of basic science, performance, side effects, and status in sports. *The American Journal of Sports Medicine*, *32*(6), 1543 1553; Yardley, J. E. & Riddell, M. C. (2016). 12 Athletes with chronic conditions. In F. Meyer, Z. Szygula & B. Wilk (eds), *Fluid Balance, Hydration, and Athletic Performance*, 265.

213 Heuberger, J. A., Cohen Tervaert, J. M., Schepers, F. M., Vliegenthart, A. D., Rotmans, J. I., Daniels, J., Burggraaf, J. & Cohen, A. F. (2013). Erythropoietin doping in cycling: Lack of evidence for efficacy and a negative risk-benefit. *British Journal of Clinical Pharmacology*, *75*(6), 1406–1421.

214 Birzniece, V. (2015). Doping in sport: Effects, harm and misconceptions. *Internal Medicine Journal*, *45*(3), 239–248.

215 Crewther, B., Obminski, Z. & Cook, C. (2016). The effect of steroid hormones on the physical performance of boys and girls during an Olympic weightlifting competition. *Pediatric Exercise Science*, *28*(4), 580–587.

216 Daughaday, W. H. & Kipnis, D. M. (2013). The growth promoting and anti-insulin actions of somatotropin. *Recent Progress in Hormone Research*, *22*, 49–99.

217 Sonksen, P. H., Cowan, D. & Holt, R. I. (2016). Use and misuse of hormones in sport. *The Lancet Diabetes & Endocrinology*, *4*(11), 882–883.

218 Handelsman, D. J. (2015). Performance enhancing hormone doping in sport. In L. Jameson, L. J. De Groot, D. M. de Krester, L. C. Giudice, A. B. Grossman, S. Melmed, J. T. Potts, . . . & W. B. Saunders (eds), *Endocrinology: Adult and Pediatric* (pp. 441–454). South Dartmouth, MA: MDText.com.

219 Nicholls, A. R. & Holt, R. I. (2016). Growth hormone and insulin-like growth factor-1. *Sports Endocrinology*, *47*, 101–114.

220 Godfrey, R. J., Madgwick, Z. & Whyte, G. P. (2003). The exercise-induced growth hormone response in athletes. *Sports Medicine*, *33*(8), 599–613.

221 Juhn, M. S. (2003). Popular sports supplements and ergogenic aids. *Sports Medicine*, *33*(12), 921–939.

222 Graham, M. R., Baker, J. S., Evans, P., Kicman, A., Cowan, D., Hullin, D., Thomas, N. & Davies, B. (2008). Physical effects of short-term recombinant human growth hormone administration in abstinent steroid dependency. *Hormone Research in Paediatrics*, *69*(6), 343–354; Graham, M. R., Davies, B., Kicman, A., Cowan, D., Hullin, D. & Baker, J. S. (2007). Recombinant human growth hormone in abstinent androgenic-anabolic steroid use: Psychological, endocrine and trophic factor effects. *Current Neurovascular Research*, *4*(1), 9–18.

223 Liu, H., Bravata, D. M., Olkin, I., Friedlander, A., Liu, V., Roberts, B., Bendavid, E., Saynina, O., Salpeter, S. R., Garber, A. M. & Hoffman, A. R. (2008). Systematic review: The effects of growth hormone on athletic performance. *Annals of Internal Medicine*, *148*(10), 747–758.

224 Meinhardt, U., Nelson, A. E., Hansen, J. L., Birzniece, V., Clifford, D., Leung, K. C., Graham, K. & Ho, K. K. (2010). The effects of growth hormone on body composition and physical performance in recreational athletesa randomized trial. *Annals of Internal Medicine*, *152*(9), 568–577.

225 Hatton, C. K., Green, G. A. & Ambrose, P. J. (2014). Performance-enhancing drugs: Understanding the risks. *Physical Medicine and Rehabilitation Clinics of North America*, *25*(4), 897–913.

226 Kicman, A. T., Brooks, R. V. & Cowan, D. A. (1991). Human chorionic gonadotrophin and sport. *British Journal of Sports Medicine*, *25*(2), 73–80.

227 Cole, L. A. (2014). *Human chorionic gonadotropin (hCG)*. Amsterdam, Netherlands: Elsevier.

228 Sansone, A., Romanelli, F., Sansone, M., Lenzi, A. & Di Luigi, L. (2017). Gyneco-mastia and hormones. *Endocrine*, *55*(1), 37–44.

229 Christou, M. A., Christou, P. A., Markozannes, G., Tsatsoulis, A., Mastorakos, G. & Tigas, S. (2017). Effects of anabolic androgenic steroids on the reproductive system of athletes and recreational users: A systematic review and meta-analysis. *Sports Medicine*, 1–15.

230 Butler, S. A. & Cole, L. A. (2016). Evidence for, and associated risks with, the Human Chorionic Gonadotropin Supplemented Diet. *Journal of Dietary Supplements*, *13*(6), 694–699.

231 Rahnema, C. D., Lipshultz, L. I., Crosnoe, L. E., Kovac, J. R. & Kim, E. D. (2014). Anabolic steroid–induced hypogonadism: Diagnosis and treatment. *Fertility and Sterility*, *101*(5), 1271–1279.

232 Russell-Jones, D. L., Umpleby, A. M., Hennessy, T., Bowes, S. B., Shojaee-Moradie, F., Hopkins, K. D., Jackson, N. C., Kelly, J. M., Jones, R. H. & Sonksen, P. H. (1994). Use of a leucine clamp to demonstrate that IGF-I actively stimulates protein synthesis in normal humans. *American Journal of Physiology–Endocrinology and Metabolism*, *267*(4), E591–E598.

233 Ip, E. J., Barnett, M. J., Tenerowicz, M. J. & Perry, P. J. (2012). Weightlifting's risky new trend: A case series of 41 insulin users. *Current Sports Medicine Reports*, *11*(4), 176–179.

234 Reverter, J. L., Tural, C., Rosell, A., Dominguez, M. & Sanmarti, A. (1994). Self-induced insulin hypoglycemia in a bodybuilder. *Archives of Internal Medicine*, *154*(2), 225–226.

235 Evans, P. J. & Lynch, R. M. (2003). Insulin as a drug of abuse in body building. *British Journal of Sports Medicine*, *37*, 356–357.

236 Giovannucci, E., Pollak, M. N., Platz, E. A., Willett, W. C., Stampfer, M. J., Majeed, N., Colditz, G. A., Speizer, F. E. & Hankinson, S. E. (2000). A prospective study of plasma insulin-like growth factor-1 and binding protein-3 and risk of colorectal neoplasia in women. *Cancer Epidemiology and Prevention Biomarkers*, *9*(4), 345–349.

237 Kicman, A. T. & Cowan, D. A. (1992). Peptide hormones and sport: misuse and detection. *British Medical Bulletin*, *48*(3), 496–517.

238 Soetens, E., Hueting, J. E. & Meirleir, K. (1995). No influence of ACTH on maximal performance. *Psychopharmacology*, *118*(3), 260–266.

239 Storer, T. W., Magliano, L., Woodhouse, L., Lee, M. L., Dzekov, C., Dzekov, J., Casaburi, R. & Bhasin, S. (2003). Testosterone dose-dependently increases maximal voluntary strength and leg power, but does not affect fatigability or specific tension. *The Journal of Clinical Endocrinology & Metabolism*, *88*(4), 1478–1485.

240 Basaria, S. (2010). Androgen abuse in athletes: detection and consequences. *The Journal of Clinical Endocrinology & Metabolism*, *95*(4), 1533–1543.

241 Vari, C. E., Ősz, B. E., Miklos, A., Berbecaruiovan, A. & Tero-Vescan, A. (2016). Aromatase inhibitors in men—off-label use, misuse, abuse and doping, *64*(6), 813–818.

242 Handelsman, D. J. (2006). The rationale for banning human chorionic gonadotropin and estrogen blockers in sport. *The Journal of Clinical Endocrinology & Metabolism*, *91*(5), 1646–1653.

243 Handelsman, D. J. (2008). Indirect androgen doping by oestrogen blockade in sports. *British Journal of Pharmacology*, *154*(3), 598–605.

244 Goss, P. E. (1999). Risks versus benefits in the clinical application of aromatase inhibitors. *Endocrine-Related Cancer*, *6*(2), 325–332.

245 Chester, N. (2014). Hormone and metabolic modulators. In D. Mottram & N. Chester (eds), *Drugs in Sport (6th edn)* (pp. 117–125). London: Routledge.

246 Dutertre, M. & Smith, C. L. (2000). Molecular mechanisms of selective estrogen receptor modulator (SERM) action. *Journal of Pharmacology and Experimental Therapeutics*, 295(2), 431–437.

247 Mazzarino, M., Braganò, M. C., de la Torre, X., Molaioni, F & Botrè, F, (2011). Relevance of the selective oestrogen receptor modulators tamoxifen, toremifene and clomiphene in doping field: endogenous steroids urinary profile after multiple oral doses. *Steroids*, 76(12), 1400–1406.

248 Nikolopoulos, D. D., Spiliopoulou, C. & Theocharis, S. E. (2011). Doping and musculoskeletal system: Short-term and long-lasting effects of doping agents. *Fundamental & Clinical Pharmacology*, 25(5), 535–563.

249 Schuelke, M., Wagner, K. R., Stolz, L. E., Hübner, C., Riebel, T., Kömen, W., Braun, T., Tobin, J. F. & Lee, S. J. (2004). Myostatin mutation associated with gross muscle hypertrophy in a child. *New England Journal of Medicine*, 350(26), 2682–2688.

250 Willoughby, D. S. (2004). Effects of an alleged myostatin-binding supplement and heavy resistance training on serum myostatin, muscle strength and mass, and body composition. *International Journal of Sport Nutrition and Exercise Metabolism*, 14(4), 461–472.

251 Matsakas, A. & Diel, P. (2005). The growth factor myostatin, a key regulator in skeletal muscle growth and homeostasis. *International Journal of Sports Medicine*, 26(2), 83–89.

252 Mosher, D. S., Quignon, P., Bustamante, C. D., Sutter, N. B., Mellersh, C. S., Parker, H. G. & Ostrander, E. A. (2007). A mutation in the myostatin gene increases muscle mass and enhances racing performance in heterozygote dogs. *PLoS Genet*, 3(5), e79–e86.

253 Prather, I. D., Brown, D. E., North, P. & Wilson, J. R. (1995). Clenbuterol: A substitute for anabolic steroids? *Medicine and Science in Sports and Exercise*, 27(8), 1118–1121.

254 Maltin, C. A., Delday, M. I., Watson, J. S., Heys, S. D., Nevison, I. M., Ritchie, I. K. & Gibson, P. H. (1993). Clenbuterol, a β-adrenoceptor agonist, increases relative muscle strength in orthopaedic patients. *Clinical Science*, 84(6), 651–654.

255 Bonetti, A., Tirelli, F., Catapano, A., Dazzi, D., Dei Cas, A., Solito, F., Ceda, G., Reverberi, C., Monica, C., Pipitone, S. & Elia, G. (2008). Side effects of anabolic androgenic steroids abuse. *International Journal of Sports Medicine*, 29(8), 679–687.

256 Nieminen, M. S., Rämö, M. P., Viitasalo, M., Heikkilä, P., Karjalainen, J., Mäntysaari, M. & Heikkila, J. (1996). Serious cardiovascular side effects of large doses of anabolic steroids in weight lifters. *European Heart Journal*, 17(10), 1576–1583.

257 Carlsen, K. H., Hem, E., Stensrud, T., Held, T., Herland, K. & Mowinckel, P. (2001). Can asthma treatment in sports be doping? The effect of the rapid onset, long-acting inhaled β2-agonist formoterol upon endurance performance in healthy well-trained athletes. *Respiratory Medicine*, 95(7), 571–576; Goubault, C., Perault, M. C., Leleu, E., Bouquet, S., Legros, P., Vandel, B. & Denjean, A. (2001). Effects of inhaled salbutamol in exercising non-asthmatic athletes. *Thorax*, 56(9), 675–679.

258 McKenzie, D. C. & Fitch, K. D. (2011). The asthmatic athlete: Inhaled Beta-2 agonists, sport performance, and doping. *Clinical Journal of Sport Medicine*, 21(1), 46–50.

259 Kindermann, W. (2007). Do inhaled b2-agonists have an ergogenic potential in non-asthmatic competitive athletes? *Sports Medicine*, 37(2), 95–102.

260 Johnson, M. (1995). Pharmacology of long-acting beta-agonists. *Annals of Allergy, Asthma & Immunology: Official Publication of the American College of Allergy, Asthma, & Immunology*, 75(2), 177–179.

261 Honour, J. W. (2016). Doping in sport: Consequences for health, clinicians and laboratories. *Annals of Clinical Biochemistry: An International Journal of Biochemistry and Laboratory Medicine*, 53(2), 189–190.

262 Brito, C. J., Roas, A. F. C. M., Brito, I. S. S., Marins, J. C. B., Córdova, C. & Franchini, E. (2012). Methods of body-mass reduction by combat sport athletes. *International Journal of Sport Nutrition and Exercise Metabolism, 22*(2), 89–97.

263 Van de Kerkhof, D. H., De Boer, D., Thijssen, J. H. & Maes, R. A. (2000). Evaluation of testosterone/epitestosterone ratio influential factors as determined in doping analysis. *Journal of Analytical Toxicology, 24*(2), 102–115.

264 Wood, R. I. & Stanton, S. J. (2012). Testosterone and sport: current perspectives. *Hormones and Behavior, 61*(1), 147–155.

265 Catlin, D. H. & Murray, T. H. (1996). Performance-enhancing drugs, fair competition, and Olympic sport. *JAMA, 276*(3), 231–237.

266 Honour, J. W. (1997). Steroid abuse in female athletes. *Current Opinion in Obstetrics and Gynecology, 9*(3), 181–186.

267 Cadwallader, A. B., De La Torre, X., Tieri, A. & Botrè, F. (2010). The abuse of diuretics as performance-enhancing drugs and masking agents in sport doping: pharmacology, toxicology and analysis. *British Journal of Pharmacology, 161*(1), 1–16.

268 Greenberg, A. (2000). Diuretic complications. *The American Journal of the Medical Sciences, 319*(1), 10–24.

269 Emran, M. A., Hossain, S. S., Salek, A. K. M., Khan, M. M., Ahmed, S. M., Khandaker, M. N. & Islam, M. T. (2014). Drug abuse in sports and doping. *Bangladesh Medical Journal, 43*(1), 46–50.

270 Avois, L., Robinson, N., Saudan, C., Baume, N., Mangin, P. & Saugy, M. (2006). Central nervous system stimulants and sport practice. *British Journal of Sports Medicine, 40*(1), i16–i20.

271 Casella, M., Russo, A. D., Izzo, G., Pieroni, M., Andreini, D., Russo, E., Colombo, D., Bologna, F., Bolognese, L., Zeppilli, P. & Tondo, C. (2015). Ventricular arrhythmias induced by long-term use of ephedrine in two competitive athletes. *Heart and Vessels, 30*(2), 280–283.

272 Abraham, J., Mudd, J. O., Kapur, N., Klein, K., Champion, H. C. & Wittstein, I. S. (2009). Stress cardiomyopathy after intravenous administration of catecholamines and beta-receptor agonists. *Journal of the American College of Cardiology, 53*(15), 1320–1325.

273 Russo, A. D., Pieroni, M., Santangeli, P., Bartoletti, S., Casella, M., Pelargonio, G., Smaldone, C., Bianco, M., Di Biase, L., Bellocci, F. & Zeppilli, P. (2011). Concealed cardiomyopathies in competitive athletes with ventricular arrhythmias and an apparently normal heart: Role of cardiac electroanatomical mapping and biopsy. *Heart Rhythm, 8*(12), 1915–1922.

274 Sagoe, D., McVeigh, J., Bjørnebekk, A., Essilfie, M. S., Andreassen, C. S. & Pallesen, S. (2015). Polypharmacy among anabolic-androgenic steroid users: a descriptive metasynthesis. *Substance Abuse Treatment, Prevention, and Policy, 10*(1), 12–31.

275 Trinh, K. V., Kim, J. & Ritsma, A. (2015). Effect of pseudoephedrine in sport: a systematic review. *BMJ Open Sport & Exercise Medicine, 1*(1), e000066–e000076.

276 Fleckenstein, A. E., Volz, T. J., Riddle, E. L., Gibb, J. W. & Hanson, G. R. (2007). New insights into the mechanism of action of amphetamines. *Annual Review of Pharmacological Toxicology, 47*, 681–698.

277 Catlin, D. H. & Hatton, C. K. (1990). Use and abuse of anabolic and other drugs for athletic enhancement. *Advances in Internal Medicine, 36*, 399–424.

278 Zaretsky, D. V., Brown, M. B., Zaretskaia, M. V., Durant, P. J. & Rusyniak, D. E. (2014). The ergogenic effect of amphetamine. *Temperature, 1*(3), 242–247.

279 Pinter, E. J. & Pattee, C. J. (1968). Fat-mobilizing action of amphetamine. *Journal of Clinical Investigation, 47*(2), 394–402.

280 Clarkson, P. M. & Thompson, H. S. (1997). Drugs and sport. *Sports Medicine, 24*(6), 366–384.

281 Dekhuijzen, P. N. R., Machiels, H. A., Heunks, L. M. A., Van der Heijden, H. F. M. & Van Balkom, R. H. H. (1999). Athletes and doping: Effects of drugs on the respiratory system. *Thorax, 54*(11), 1041–1046.

282 Piţigoi, G., Păunescu, C., Petrescu, S., Ciolan, G. A. & Păunescu, M. (2013). Drug abuse in sport performance—A systematic review, *Farmacia*, *61*(6), 1037–1042.

283 De Jonge, R., Bolt, I., Schermer, M. & Olivier, B. (2008). Botox for the brain: Enhancement of cognition, mood and pro-social behavior and blunting of unwanted memories. *Neuroscience and Biobehavioral Reviews*, *32*, 760–776.

284 Franke, A. G. Gransmark, P. Agricola, A., Schuhle, K., Rommel, T., Sebastian, A, Ballo H. E., Gorbulev, S., Gerdes, C., Frank, B., Ruckes, C., Tuscher, O. & Lieb, K. (2017). Methylphenidate, modafinil, and caffeine for cognitive enhancement in chess: A double-blind, randomised controlled trial. *European Neuropsychopharmacology*, *27*(3) 248–260. http://dx.doi.org/10.1016/j.euroneuro.2017.01.006

285 de Jonge, R., Bolt, I., Schermer, M. & Olivier, B. (2008). Botox for the brain: Enhancement of cognition, mood and pro-social behavior and blunting of unwanted memories. *Neuroscience and Biobehavioral Reviews*, *32*, 760–776.

286 Franke, A. G., Bonertz, C., Christmann, M., Huss, M., Fellgiebel, A. Hildt, E. & Lieb, K. (2010). Non-medical use of prescription stimulants and illicit use of stimulents for cognitive enhancement in pupils and students in Germany. *Pharmacopsychiatry*, *44*, 60–66.

287 Smith, M. E. & Farah, M. J. (2011). Are prescription stimulants "smart pills"?: The epidemiology and cognitive neuroscience of prescription stimulant use by normal healthy individuals. *Psychological Bulletin*, *137*(5), 717–741.

288 Repantis, D., Schlattmann, P. Laisney, O. & Heuser, I. (2010). Modafinil and methylphenidate for neuroenhancment in healthy individuals: A systematic review. *Pharmacological Research*, *62*, 187–206.

289 Lakhan, S. E. & Kirschgessner, A. (2012). Prescription stimulants in individuals with and without attention deficit hyperactivity disorder: Misuse, cognitive impact, and adverse effects. *Brain and Behavior*, *2*(5), 661–677.

290 Frati, P., Kyriakou, C., Del Rio, A., Marinelli, E., Vergallo, G. M., Zami, S. & Busardò, F. P. (2015). Smart drugs and synthetic androgens for cognitive and physical enhancement: Revolving doors of cosmetic neurology. *Current Neuropharmacology*, *13*(1), 5–11.

291 Smith, M. E. & Farah, M. J. (2011). Are prescription stimulants "smart pills"?: The epidemiology and cognitive neuroscience of prescription stimulant use by normal healthy individuals. *Psychological Bulletin*, *137*(5), 717–741.

292 De Jonge, R., Bolt, I., Schermer, M. & Olivier, B. (2008). Botox for the brain: Enhancement of cognition, mood and pro-social behavior and blunting of unwanted memories. *Neuroscience and Biobehavioral Reviews*, *32*, 760–776.

293 de Jonge, R., Bolt, I., Schermer, M. & Olivier, B. (2008). Botox for the brain: Enhancement of cognition, mood and pro-social behavior and blunting of unwanted memories. *Neuroscience and Biobehavioral Reviews*, *32*, 760–776.

294 Franke, A. G., Gransmark, P., Agricola, A., Schuhle, K., Rommel, T., Sebastian, A., Ballo H. E., Gorbulev, S., Gerdes, C., Frank, B., Ruckes, C., Tuscher, O. & Lieb, K. (2017). Methylphenidate, modafinil, and caffeine for cognitive enhancement in chess: A double-blind, randomised controlled trial. *European Neuropsychopharmacology*, *27*(3) 248–260. http://dx.doi.org/10.1016/j.euroneuro.2017.01.006

295 Repantis, D., Schlattmann, P. Laisney, O. & Heuser, I. (2010). Modafinil and methylphenidate for neuroenhancment in healthy individuals: A systematic review. *Pharmacological Research*, *62*, 187–206.

296 Repantis, D., Schlattmann, P. Laisney, O. & Heuser, I. (2010). Modafinil and methylphenidate for neuroenhancment in healthy individuals: A systematic review. *Pharmacological Research*, *62*, 187–206.

297 Copani, A., Genazzani, A. A., Aleppo, G., Casabona, G., Canonico, P. L., Scapagnini, U. & Nicoletti, F. (1992). Nootropic drugs positively modulate α-amino-3-hydroxy-5-methyl-4-isoxazolepropionic acid-sensitive glutamate receptors in neuronal cultures. *Journal of Neurochemistry*, *58*, 1199–1204.

298 Giurgea, C. E. (1982). The nootropic concept and its prospective implications. *Drug Development Research*, *2*, 441–446.

299 Villardita, C., Grioli S., Lomeo, C., Cattane, C. & Parini, J. (1992). Clinical studies with oxiracetam in patients with dementia of Alzheimer type and multi-infarct dementia of mild to moderate degree. *Neuropsychobiology*, *25*, 24–28.

300 Lee, C. R. & Benfield, P. (1994). Aniracetam. An overview of its pharmacodynamic and pharmacokinetic properties, and a review of its therapeutic potential in senile cognitive disorders. *Drugs & Aging*, *4*, 257–273.

301 Parnetti, L., Mecocci, P., Petrini, A., Longo, A., Buccolieri, A. & Senin, U. (1989). Neuropsychological results of long-term therapy with oxiracetam in patients with dementia of Alzheimer type and multi-infarct dementia in comparison with a control group. *Neuropsychobiology*, *22*, 97–100.

302 Julien, R. M., Advokat, C. D. & Comaty, J. E. (2008). *A Primer of Drug Action (11th edn)*. New York: Worth Publishers.

303 MacAuley, D. (1996). Drugs in sport. *British Medical Journal*, *313*(7051), 211–215.

304 Emran, M. A., Hossain, S. S., Salek, A. K. M., Khan, M. M., Ahmed, S. M., Khandaker, M. N. & Islam, M. T. (2014). Drug abuse in sports and doping. *Bangladesh Medical Journal*, *43*(1), 46–50.

305 Denham, B. E. (2014). High school sports participation and substance use: Differences by sport, race, and gender. *Journal of Child & Adolescent Substance Abuse*, *23*(3), 145–154.

306 Cicero, T. J., Ellis, M. S. & Harney, J. (2015). Shifting patterns of prescription opioid and heroin abuse in the United States. *New England Journal of Medicine*, *373*(18), 1789–1790.

307 Veliz, P., Boyd, C. J. & McCabe, S. E. (2017). Nonmedical use of prescription opioids and heroin use among adolescents involved in competitive sports. *Journal of Adolescent Health*, *60*(3), 346–349.

308 Benedetti, F., Pollo, A. & Colloca, L. (2007). Opioid-mediated placebo responses boost pain endurance and physical performance: Is it doping in sport competitions? *Journal of Neuroscience*, *27*(44), 11934–11939.

309 De Jong, G., Maes, R. A. A. & Van Rossum, J. M. (1988). Doping control of athletes. *Trends in Analytical Chemistry*, *7*(10), 375–382.

310 Dvorak, J., Graf-Baumann, T., D'Hooghe, M., Kirkendall, D., Taennler, H. & Saugy, M. (2006). FIFA's approach to doping in football. *British Journal of Sports Medicine*, *40*(1), i3–i12.

311 Mauger, A. R., Taylor, L., Bryna, C., Chrismas, R., Watkins, S. L. & Foster, J. (2014). Reply to letter: Acetaminophen and sport performance: doping or what? *European Journal of Applied Physiology*, *114*(4), 883–884.

312 Veliz, P. T., Boyd, C. & McCabe, S. E. (2013). Playing through pain: Sports participation and nonmedical use of opioid medications among adolescents. *American Journal of Public Health*, *103*(5), e28–e30.

313 Smuin, D. M., Seidenberg, P. H., Sirlin, E. A., Phillips, S. F. & Silvis, M. L. (2016). Rare adverse events associated with corticosteroid injections: A case series and literature review. *Current Sports Medicine Reports*, *15*(3), 171–176.

314 Orchard, J. W. (2017). Systematic review is the highest level of evidence for knee osteoarthritis injection options, not expert society guidelines. *British Journal of Sports Medicine*, *51*(7), 622–622.

315 Krogh, T. P., Bartels, E. M., Ellingsen, T., Stengaard-Pedersen, K., Buchbinder, R., Fredberg, U., Bliddal, H. & Christensen, R. (2013). Comparative effectiveness of injection therapies in lateral epicondylitis: A systematic review and network meta-analysis of randomized controlled trials. *The American Journal of Sports Medicine*, *41*(6), 1435–1446.

316 Ranalletta, M., Rossi, L. A., Bongiovanni, S. L., Tanoira, I., Elizondo, C. M. & Maignon, G. D. (2016). Corticosteroid injections accelerate pain relief and recovery of function compared with oral NSAIDs in patients with adhesive capsulitis: A randomized controlled trial. *The American Journal of Sports Medicine*, *44*(2), 474–481.

317 Drakos, M., Birmingham, P., Delos, D., Barnes, R., Murphy, C., Weiss, L. & Warren, R. (2014). Corticosteroid and anesthetic injections for muscle strains and ligament sprains in the NFL. *HSS Journal(r)*, *10*(2), 136–142.

318 Smuin, D. M., Seidenberg, P. H., Sirlin, E. A., Phillips, S. F. & Silvis, M. L. (2016). Rare adverse events associated with corticosteroid injections: A case series and literature review. *Current Sports Medicine Reports, 15*(3), 171–176.

319 Maman, E., Yehuda, C., Pritsch, T., Morag, G., Brosh, T., Sharfman, Z. & Dolkart, O. (2016). Detrimental effect of repeated and single subacromial corticosteroid injections on the intact and injured rotator cuff: A biomechanical and imaging study in rats. *The American Journal of Sports Medicine*, *44*(1), 177–182.

320 Desai, S., Aldea, D., Daneels, E., Soliman, M., Braksmajer, A. S. & Kopes-Kerr, C. P. (2006). Chronic addiction to dextromethorphan cough syrup: a case report. *The Journal of the American Board of Family Medicine*, *19*(3), 320–323.

321 Wax, P. M. (2002). Just a click away: Recreational drug web sites on the Internet. *Pediatrics*, *109*(6), e96–e96.

322 Agnich, L. E., Stogner, J. M., Miller, B. L. & Marcum, C. D. (2013). Purple drink prevalence and characteristics of misusers of codeine cough syrup mixtures. *Addictive Behaviors*, *38*(9), 2445–2449.

323 Lessenger, J. E. & Feinberg, S. D. (2008). Abuse of prescription and over-the-counter medications. *The Journal of the American Board of Family Medicine*, *21*(1), 45–54.

324 Bianco, A., Thomas, E., Pomara, F., Tabacchi, G., Karsten, B., Paoli, A. & Palma, A. (2014). Alcohol consumption and hormonal alterations related to muscle hypertrophy: A review. *Nutrition & Metabolism*, *11*(1), 26–34.

325 Reardon, C. L. & Creado, S. (2014). Drug abuse in athletes. *Substance Abuse Rehabilitation*, *5*, 95–105.

326 Davis, E., Loiacono, R. & Summers, R. J. (2008). The rush to adrenaline: drugs in sport acting on the β-adrenergic system. *British Journal of Pharmacology*, *154*(3), 584–597.

327 Davis, E., Loiacono, R. & Summers, R. J. (2008). The rush to adrenaline: drugs in sport acting on the β-adrenergic system. *British Journal of Pharmacology*, *154*(3), 584–597.

328 Kruse, P., Ladefoged, J., Nielsen, U., Paulev, P. E. & Sorensen, J. P. (1986). Beta-blockade used in precision sports: Effect on pistol shooting performance. *Journal of Applied Physiology*, *61*(2), 417–420.

329 Creado, S. & Reardon, C. (2016). The sports psychiatrist and performance-enhancing drugs. *International Review of Psychiatry*, *28*(6), 564–571.

330 Head, A., Kendall, M. J., Ferner, R. & Eagles, C. (1996). Acute effects of beta blockade and exercise on mood and anxiety. *British Journal of Sports Medicine*, *30*(3), 238–242.

331 Dimsdale, J. E. & Newton, R. P. (1989). Neuropsychological side effects of β-blockers. *Archives of Internal Medicine*, *149*(3), 514–525.

332 Gordon, N. F. & Duncan, J. J. (1991). Effect of beta-blockers on exercise physiology: Implications for exercise training. *Medicine and Science in Sports and Exercise*, *23*(6), 668–676.

333 Huestis, M. A., Mazzoni, I. & Rabin, O. (2011). Cannabis in sport. *Sports Medicine*, *41*(11), 949–966.

334 Saugy, M., Avois, L., Saudan, C., Robinson, N., Giroud, C., Mangin, P. & Dvorak, J. (2006). Cannabis and sport. *British Journal of Sports Medicine*, *40*(1), i13–i15.

335 Campos, D. R., Yonamine, M. & de Moraes Moreau, R. L. (2003). Marijuana as doping in sports. *Sports Medicine*, *33*(6), 395–399.

336 Kennedy, M. C. (2017). Cannabis: exercise performance and sport. A systematic review. *Journal of Science and Medicine in Sport*, dx.doi.org/10.1016/j.jsams.2017.03.012.

337 Tacey, A., Parker, L., Garnham, A., Brennan-Speranza, T. C. & Levinger, I. (2017). The effect of acute and short term glucocorticoid administration on exercise capacity and metabolism. *Journal of Science and Medicine in Sport*, doi.org/10.1016/j.jsams.2016.10.016.

338 Zorgati, H., Prieur, F., Vergniaud, T., Cottin, F., Do, M. C., Labsy, Z., Amarantini, D., Gagey, O., Lasne, F. & Collomp, K. (2014). Ergogenic and metabolic effects of oral glucocorticoid intake during repeated bouts of high-intensity exercise. *Steroids*, *86*, 10–15.

339 Casuso, R. A., Melskens, L., Bruhn, T., Secher, N. H. & Nordsborg, N. B. (2014). Glucocorticoids improve high-intensity exercise performance in humans. *European Journal of Applied Physiology*, *114*(2), 419–424.

340 Duclos, M. (2010). Evidence on ergogenic action of glucocorticoids as a doping agent risk. *The Physician and Sportsmedicine*, *38*(3), 121–127.

341 Rafacho, A., Ortsäter, H., Nadal, A. & Quesada, I. (2014). Glucocorticoid treatment and endocrine pancreas function: implications for glucose homeostasis, insulin resistance and diabetes. *Journal of Endocrinology*, *223*(3), R49–R62.

342 Peckett, A. J., Wright, D. C. & Riddell, M. C. (2011). The effects of glucocorticoids on adipose tissue lipid metabolism. *Metabolism*, *60*(11), 1500–1510.

343 Oray, M., Abu Samra, K., Ebrahimiadib, N., Meese, H. & Foster, C. S. (2016). Long-term side effects of glucocorticoids. *Expert Opinion on Drug Safety*, *15*(4), 457–465.

344 Rotunno, A., van Rensburg, D. J., Grant, C. C. & van Rensburg, A. J. (2016). Corticosteroids in sports-related injuries: Friend or Foe. *South African Family Practice*, *58*(6), 28–33.

345 Handelsman, D. J. (2015). Performance enhancing hormone doping in sport. In L. Jameson, L. J. De Groot, D. M. de Krester, L. C. Giudice, A. B. Grossman, S. Melmed, J. T. Potts, . . . & W. B. Saunders (eds), *Endocrinology: Adult and Pediatric* (pp. 441–454). South Dartmouth, MA: MDText.com.

7

GIVENS, GAPS, CONFIDENCES AND CAUTIONS

Conclusion

Introduction: A growth industry

PIEDS of all kinds occupy a crucially important, but awkward space, in contemporary society. They have become a pivotal component of good medical care, they improve people's quality of life, they give people intense—if sometimes only ephemeral—pleasure, they augment athletic performance and they enable others to extend their lifespans. PIEDS of all kinds are used across the human life-course, with every age cohort securing comfort and relief from a bevy of substances.

When DNS and over-the-counter medicines are included, it is clear that most people in developed nations use PIEDS regularly. While some substances are misused, and produce significant social costs, they also provide people with respite from chronic pain, allow them to manage a disability more effectively, make their lives more manageable and in many cases make their lives more pleasurable. In addition, recreational and elite athletes in every sport and leisure activity conduct their daily lives in a wider world where PIEDS use is embedded in culture and practice.

In short, there is widespread dependence on PIEDS to help people cope with the pressures and tensions of their daily lives, making them feel psychologically confident and physically better. PIEDS use is clearly not an aberrant behaviour confined to a problematic subculture of deviants and misfits, but rather a common practice amongst the mainstream population. However, PIEDS, especially for males, provides a mechanism whereby users can play out their ideals of masculinity and manhood. In this context, PIEDS become part of the playing-out process, since they not only feed the need to compete and win, but also feed the need to engage in high-risk behaviour. In these instances, failure, defeat, injury and even social stigma and shame, are not problems provided they are associated with heroic outcomes. Equally, many females feel compelled to take PIEDS in order to comply with socially constructed views of femininity. Although an immensely complex area, our review of PIEDS in this book has revealed some critical themes, which are summarised next.

Summary of key points

The supply of PIEDS has proliferated, offering something for every imaginable physical objective, whether muscle building and fat burning, or to combat inflammation and bolster joint health. A growing supply of so-called smart drugs for cognitive enhancement will shortly join the list as their reputation grows and their availability improves.

This book defines PIEDS as any material an individual enters into (through ingestion or injection), or applies on the surface of his or her body, to enhance physical performance or appearance as well as cognitive functioning. Included are pharmaceutical drugs (prescription, e.g. amphetamines; over-the-counter, e.g. alcohol, analgesics, caffeine; illicit, e.g. cocaine) and dietary or nutritional supplements (e.g. amino acids). Also included are substances athletes use for recreational, recovery or stress-management purposes, and which may be perceived as indirectly performance enhancing. PIEDS further encompass any substance used for augmenting aesthetic bodily appearance, but exclude cosmetics and 'cosmeceuticals' applied to the skin.

While the premises that sport's capacity to 1) build character, 2) channel the energies of its participants into constructive social activities and 3) guide its participants into naturalistic and healthy lifestyles receive wide acceptance, the evidence in support of these claims is hardly conclusive. For the most part, the studies reviewed here indicate that people who play sport, regularly hang around sport clubs and use gyms to build their bodies do actually use PIEDS and other substances more often that those who do other things with their spare time. The seminal longitudinal study by Peck et al., which followed US adolescents through to adulthood, confirmed this proposition.[1] That is to say, sport participation as an adolescent does not of itself lead to increased PIEDS use, but when combined with 1) sport as a central life focus, 2) a preference for broader drug use and 3) aggressive attitudes to their social worlds, there is a tight correspondence with high levels of PIEDS and related substance use, especially alcohol consumption.

Overall, there is sufficient evidence to confidently claim that PIEDS use—be it prescription, over the counter or illicit—takes place in all sorts of sport and physical recreation settings around the world. The work of the Australian Crime Commission,[2] the Australian Institute of Health and Welfare[3] and researchers such as Alaranta et al.[4] have illuminated its causes, consequences and diffusion. It occurs in school sport, although most of the data discussed in this book applied to American high schools where inter-school sport is highly valued, and where it contributes significantly to a school's reputation and financial viability. PIEDS use also seems prevalent in community gyms and fitness centres, with Europe and the US featuring prominently in the research findings. PIEDS appear liberally in colleges and universities as well, where American studies show that both licit and illicit substance use is usually higher amongst athletes than non-athletes. Finally, PIEDS use in all its guises is clearly a common practice in not only elite and professional sport, but also in community sport, especially where strength, endurance and good pain management constitute key success factors.

Most disappointingly, there is no evidence to suggest that unguided PIEDS use in sport or for image purposes will diminish any time soon. In fact, when substance use is expanded to cover dietary and nutritional supplement consumption—including caffeine—then the usage rates increase exponentially.[5] Within this exceedingly broad definition of PIEDS use in sport, it would be reasonable to think that more than 90% of all people have used some form of supplement, drug or related substance to get a physical or mental advantage at some time in their lives.

A major part of the PIEDS challenge is that thousands of products are available, ranging from the most commonplace multivitamin to the most exotic herbal extract, with the most potent pharmaceutical compound available through conventional prescriptions but also through unregulated online sources. In addition, some PIEDS enjoy considerable scientific validation, some are demonstrably ineffectual, some are potentially deleterious to health, some are remarkably and almost instantaneously effective and most show either a trivial effect or no effect at all, or have not been studied sufficiently to merit a confident declaration one way or another.[6]

To make matters more complicated for consumers, PIEDS manufacturers soak the cluttered marketplace with aggressive advertising proclaiming radical results alongside sponsored athletes, who not only advocate for the products, but attribute their carved and curved bodies to seemingly 'too good to be true' promises. Yet, the belligerent marketing seems to work.[7] Amongst all of the slick, pharmaceutically inspired labels, implausible body imagery, remarkable claims, safety assurances and prices bulging even more than the display models, consumers tend to believe that PIEDS work, and for the most part are unaware that little evidence underpins their veracity or that few regulatory standards guarantee quality, potency and purity.

Consumers collectively spend billions on PIEDS to bolster energy,[8] build muscle, strength and endurance,[9] attenuate fatigue,[10] facilitate recovery,[11] offset deficiencies and avoid or repair illness and generally sustain greater health.[12] In fact, the use of PIEDS—especially in the form of supplements—is not only considered routine, but also a sound and intelligent strategy for performance or cosmetic enhancement.[13]

In this book, we identified 10 major issues emerging from the available research on PIEDS. These points are summarised in Table 7.1.

Finally, we provide two further illustrations to assist in summarising PIEDS types and usages. Table 7.2 presents a typology of PIEDS based on their performance effects. In the table, substance performance has been divided into four levels of probable affect, from performance-reduction at one extreme to performance enhancement at the other. Substance access is divided into four categories, comprising illicit, prescription, over-the-counter and supplements.

TABLE 7.1 Summary of main points	
No.	Summary point
1	The abuse of some PIEDS can have serious, deleterious implications upon the long-term health of users, both during active use and well after use has discontinued.
2	The use of PIEDS exclusively for image enhancing purposes now exceeds PIEDS use for either sporting performance or medical interventions.
3	Most PIEDS usage is moderate, but the pathological and supra-therapeutic use of substances, dosages and combinations has become normalised in some communities.
4	PIEDS users obtain a significant amount of their knowledge and advice about substances, effects, dosages and distribution through unreliable online sources.
5	The authenticity, quality and potential contamination of PIEDS products have become worrisome.
6	The majority of pharmaceutical-grade PIEDS are acquired without medical guidance or a prescription.
7	Driving forces behind PIEDS use are gender associations, dysfunctional body images and a powerful desire to meet cultural ideals of health and image.
8	More effective programmes for changing attitudes, behaviours or intentions relating to PIEDS deliver over longer periods, comprise numerous teaching sessions, address a range of topics including drug- and alcohol-related issues and alternatives to drug use and media/peer pressure resistance, and increase participant involvement and ownership through peer-led teaching.
9	Emerging evidence links PIEDS abuse with gateway behaviours, beginning with DNS and moving into PEDS.
10	There remains a great deal of confusion about the effects, veracity, risks and legality of different PIEDS.

TABLE 7.2 A performance-based typology of PIEDS

		Performance reduction	Performance neutral	Performance maintenance	Performance enhancement
Ease of access	Illicit	Heroin	Marijuana	MDMAs (Ecstasy)	Amphetamines Cocaine
	Prescription	Barbiturates	Selective serotonin re-uptake inhibitors (SSRIs) (anti-depressants)	Antibiotics	Beta-blockers Androgenic anabolic steroids (AAS) Erythropoietin
	Over-the-counter	Alcohol	Nicotine	Analgesics	Caffeine Stimulants
	Supplements	Calorie-blockers Aphrodisiacs	Fat burners Vitamins Minerals	Fish oil Curcumin Glucosamine	Proteins Creatine Energy drinks Carbohydrates
		Contribution to performance enhancement			

Conclusion

Despite concerted attempts—through both regulation and education—to control and direct PIEDS use, all of the evidence indicates that use has radically increased. In fact, it points to the spread of PIEDS use from the esoteric world of elite professional sport to the commonplace world of personal appearance.

There are a number of reasons for the upward trend. A core factor has to do with the use of substances to not only enhance athletic performance, but also to improve physical appearance. An additional factor has to do with the creative use of prescription drugs and medicines to better manage pain, reduce tissue inflammation, improve endurance, focus attention and alleviate stress and anxiety. In addition, the contamination of dietary and nutritional substances with banned substances contributes to an increase in inadvertent use.

These problems are compounded by the intensive online promotion of all sorts of products that come with exaggerated claims about the efficacy and enhancement capabilities of PIEDS. The situation becomes even more complicated when decisions to use are based on part-truths, hearsay and the testimonials of players and gym users with limited knowledge about the pharmacological properties of their preferred substances.

Despite performance and health benefits accompanying the use of many legal supplements and substances, the limited available evidence suggests that some people use more and riskier PIEDS as they move through their life courses. A little PIEDS use seems to lead to more, which in turn leads to more dangerous, and sometimes illicit or banned, PIEDS. Yet, we know little about the pathways facilitating this escalation in use, or the decision-making that underpins the choices elite and recreational athletes make at each stage of their competitive life courses and their corresponding image expectations.

Performance and image enhancing drugs and substances are currently out of control, and if left unregulated and mismanaged are likely to damage the health and well-being of millions of people of all ages. The time for action on this front has arrived, and it begins with better information, education and regulation.

Notes

1 Peck, S., Vida, M. & Eccles, S. (2008). Adolescent pathways to adulthood drinking: sport activity involvement is not necessarily risky or protective. *Addiction*, *103*(1), 69–83.
2 Australian Crime Commission (2013). *Organised Crime and Drugs in Sport: New Generation Performance and Image Enhancement Drugs and Organised Criminal Involvement in Their Use in Professional Sport*. Canberra: Commonwealth of Australia.
3 Australian Institute of Health and Welfare (2008). 2007 National drug strategy household Survey: First results. Drug statistics series 20. Canberra: AIHW.
4 Alaranta, A., Alaranta, H., Holmila, J., Palmu, P., Pietilä, K. & Helenius, I. (2006). Self-reported attitudes of elite athletes towards doping: Differences between type of sport. *International Journal of Sports Medicine*, *27*, 842–846.
5 Bojsen-Moller, A. & Christiansen, A. (2010). Use of performance and image enhancing substances among recreational athletes: a quantitative analysis of inquiries submitted to

the Danish anti-doping authorities. *Scandinavian Journal of Medicine and Science in Sports*, *20*, 861–867.

6 Raja, R. R. (2016). Nutraceuticals and cosmeceuticals for human beings—An overview. *American Journal of Food Science and Health*, *2*(2), 7–17.

7 Bolton, L. E., Reed, A., Volpp, K. G. & Armstrong, K. (2008). How does drug and supplement marketing affect a healthy lifestyle? *Journal of Consumer Research*, *34*(5), 713–726.

8 Erdman, K. A., Fung, T. S., Doyle-Baker, P. K., Verhoef, M. J. & Reimer, R. A. (2007). Dietary supplementation of high-performance Canadian athletes by age and gender. *Clinical Journal of Sport Medicine*, *17*(6), 458–464.

9 Petróczi, A., Naughton, D. P., Mazanov, J., Holloway, A. & Bingham, J. (2007). Performance enhancement with supplements: incongruence between rationale and practice. *Journal of the International Society of Sports Nutrition*, *4*(1), 19.

10 Laure, P. & Binsinger, C. (2005). Adolescent athletes and the demand and supply of drugs to improve their performance. *Journal of Sports Science and Medicine*, *4*(3), 272–277.

11 Laure, P. & Binsinger, C. (2005). Adolescent athletes and the demand and supply of drugs to improve their performance. *Journal of Sports Science and Medicine*, *4*(3), 272–277.

12 Erdman, K. A., Fung, T. S., Doyle-Baker, P. K., Verhoef, M. J. & Reimer, R. A. (2007). Dietary supplementation of high-performance Canadian athletes by age and gender. *Clinical Journal of Sport Medicine*, *17*(6), 458–464.

13 Laos, C. & Metzl, J. D. (2006). Performance-enhancing drug use in young athletes. *Adolescent Medicine Clinics*, *17*(3), 719–731; Maughan, R. J., Depiesse, F. & Geyer, H. (2007). The use of dietary supplements by athletes. *Journal of Sports Sciences*, *25*(S1), S103–S113.

INDEX

Page numbers in *italics* refer to figures. Page numbers in **bold** refer to tables.

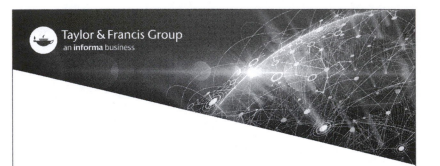